PL Y BETTER G MES

Carmel Conn

Enabling children with autism to join in with everyday games

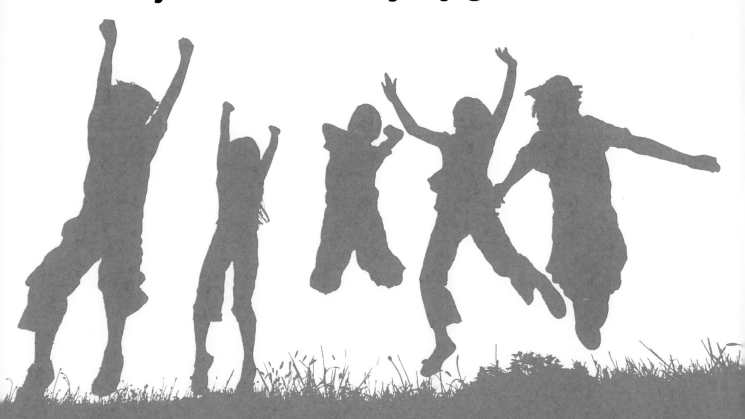

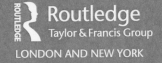

Routledge
Taylor & Francis Group

LONDON AND NEW YORK

First published 2010 by Speechmark Publishing Ltd.

Published 2017 by Routledge
2 Park Square, Milton Park, Abingdon, Oxon OX14 4RN
711 Third Avenue, New York, NY 10017, USA

Routledge is an imprint of the Taylor & Francis Group, an informa business

ISBN: 9780863888212 (pbk)

Contents

List of games

Cooperation

Rhythmic games

Games of togetherness

Looking and finding games

Self-regulation

Games of exertion

Games that focus attention

Exciting games

Adapting to others

Mutual enjoyment through games

Games that avoid conflict

Games with rules

Creativity

Preface

Many children with autism want to join in with the social play of other children, but do not know how. *Play Better Games* aims to provide ways of supporting those children with autism who do want to play more with other children. It provides enjoyable games that are better suited to groups of children who are mixed in terms of playing ability. It outlines simpler versions of more complicated games and gives a structured approach to facilitating the skills needed to take part in ordinary playground games. *Play Better Games* emphasises the need to help children be more aware of what skills are required when playing games as well as have the chance to practise and develop some of those skills for themselves.

Ordinary games are an important vehicle for children's learning. They provide a powerful, naturally occurring learning environment that is physical, playful and fun. Playing games requires interpersonal skills in language, thought, social behaviour, creativity, self-regulation and skilful use of the body. When children play games together they develop the following key capacities:

• cooperative behaviour

• focused attention

• social understanding

• holding information in mind

• motor, spatial and sequential planning

• self-regulation, eg impulse control, coping with excitement, controlled exertion

• collaborative behaviour and negotiation

• self-expression and creativity.

Games fulfil the requirement that learning should be embodied, enjoyable and adaptable to the needs of all. Games provide a social experience that is emotionally compelling, where children laugh and have fun and do not even realise they are interacting, problem solving, negotiating and cooperating with each other.

Many children with autism want to take part in games but are prohibited by the sheer sophistication of the social, cognitive and communicative skills required. Skills are often combined in games, making the playing even more challenging. In addition, the motor skill involved in many games – playing with balls, running and dodging, coordinated physical play – can be highly prohibitive. Challenge exists too in other areas of playing games: in the generation of narratives, for example, or the need to adapt one's interests in play to the interests of others.

Some children with autism enjoy playing a game but do not move on in terms of play skill. Young children with autism often love to be chased but may never allow themselves to be caught. Such children may benefit from having clear visual boundaries marked out in a game. Other children may need help to understand the ordinary conventions of play and friendship.

They may appreciate being told, for example, that conflict is most common among friends and is something most people find hard to deal with.

In supporting children with autism, we are often challenged in our knowledge and understanding, forced to think more deeply about what goes on socially and cognitively for all children. Working through games with children on the autism spectrum is no exception. In order to facilitate access to ordinary games, we need to think about what skills a game involves and consider how we can develop or support these.

Play Better Games is designed to help practitioners and parents to think about what might prohibit their child from joining in with games and to plan effective strategies for support. It will be of benefit to teachers, therapists, group workers, play workers, midday supervisors and support workers, as well as to parents and siblings of children with autism. Many of the games that are included here will be familiar. What is given special attention is the particular skills needed to play a game, with the emphasis on gradually developing an ability to play more skilful games.

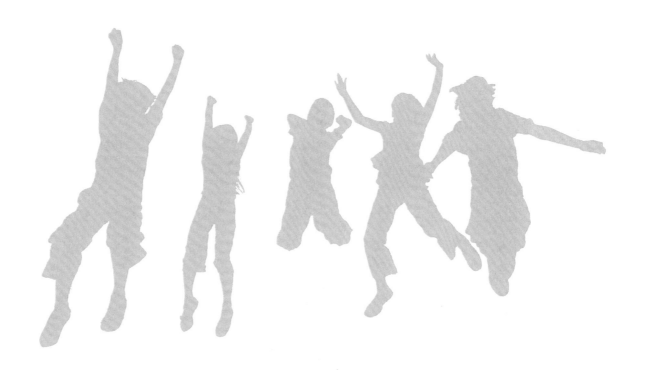

How to use this book

Play Better Games is for use with primary age children in schools, play schemes and group settings as well as at home. It is designed in a simple and straightforward manner to give ideas on how to support children with autism to interact and play with other children. The games described here could be used at playtimes, during PSHE, in circle time, in small group work, indoors or in the park. It is for use with children with autism who want to join in with games wherever they are being played. *Play Better Games* takes a developmental approach, beginning with early forms of interaction, using simple reciprocity and cooperation, and moving on to more sophisticated games that involve social adjustment, negotiation, creativity and pretence.

The four areas of development are:

• playing cooperatively with others

• regulating one's feelings, attention and impulses

• adapting to others' needs and interests

• creativity in playing games.

Within each of these four areas, games are organised into discrete areas of learning:

• **cooperation**
  - games that involve simple taking turns
  - games that promote a shared enjoyment of being together
  - looking for people and taking pleasure in finding them

• **self-regulation**
  - strength games that require controlled physical and mental exertion
  - games that help to organise attention
  - exciting games that require dealing with strong feelings and impulses

• **adapting to others**
  - games that give an experience of having fun in a group
  - learning how to avoid conflict in games
  - playing games with rules

• **creativity**
  - games that require physical, facial and dramatic expression
  - making up stories in games
  - pretending, improvising and thinking up new games.

So often in autism education, social skills learning is taken out of the context of children's everyday lives and has little connection with how they really interact with one another. It is probable that many of the skills needed for interpersonal engagement, friendship and play can only be acquired within the actual context of everyday interactions. The focus here is on enabling children with autism to play specific games with other children so that, through playing games, skills can be tried out. The skill areas that are supported here are ones that are relevant both to the social needs of children with autism and to what children really do when playing with each other. Above all, children should have a good and satisfying experience of being together as a way of building social confidence and relationships.

In the spirit of children's games, the games described here are highly adaptive. Most of them can be played with a small number of children or with a larger group; many can be played outdoors or indoors. The games can be used with mixed groups of children, and children of different ages and with differing levels of ability. They require little or no equipment, only everyday objects that are readily to hand.

The social impairment in autism is, to some extent, a shared impairment. Interventions often require learning on the part of the individual with autism as well as for those around them, with misunderstanding often occurring on both sides. *Play Better Games* takes a dual approach, offering ways of supporting children with autism while also providing explanations and information that might be useful to teachers, parents and children without autism.

For this purpose, each chapter has:

• an **introduction** to the area of learning covered in that chapter

• a list of **key terms** which can be shared with all children and discussed to aid their understanding of the particular social issue

• a **progression of skills** involved in playing the games in each chapter

• a **'Think About' discussion** which focuses on common areas of difficulty within play, such as winning and losing and being 'It'. 'Think About' discussions give an adult-oriented explanation of the issues involved. Simpler explanations and suggestions for children are also included to develop their understanding.

Play Better Games is not designed as a heavily prescriptive programme of work, but rather a support that can be dipped into for ideas and information. It is not expected that all children will be able to join in with all the games here. Some children with autism will not be able to access the more sophisticated games. However, many will and the idea is that they can be enabled to play more difficult games by practising the skills needed for them in simpler but related games. *Play Better Games* can be used as a way of considering what games a child can presently access as well as facilitating the capacity to play other related games.

Cooperation

Cooperation is used here to refer to social interaction that is reciprocal and provides a satisfying social experience for those involved. In the games that follow, moving together in a coordinated and cooperative way will be important, as will working towards social exchange that has a rhythmic back and forth quality. Above all, these games are about finding enjoyment in other people's company, having fun together, showing pleasure in finding someone and feeling that one is being appreciated by others.

Cooperation

1 Rhythmic games

These games play with the idea that interaction has a rhythm to it, a back and forth, first then second, me then you sequence. The rhythms used here are kept simple since it is often hard for children with autism to join in with the rhythm of an interaction, often needing a little more time to take their turn. However, the simple structures of these games should give a good experience of rhythm in interaction and enable children to practise taking their turn.

The first two games involve repeating a simple social activity with a small variation each time. The next games focus on taking turns in a game, through call and response techniques and through the physical actions of throwing a ball and jumping over a partner. The final five games require more in the way of skill on the part of players, but retain a strong rhythmic element, using a back and forth, up and down or side to side action in the play.

Key terms

repeating, taking turns, tick-tock

Progression of skills

• repeat an activity with slight variation

• take turns in a group

• carry out a physical activity in a coordinated way

• move rhythmically.

5-4-3-2-1!

This is a lively group activity with a strong and simple rhythm.

Organisation of players

Players stand in a circle.

Playing the game

1 Altogether, players stamp their feet in rhythm and punch their fists alternately in the air.

2 Once a rhythm has been established and continuing to stamp and punch their fists, players chant 'Five-four-three-two-one-____' in rhythm with their feet and call out the name of someone in the circle.

3 This is repeated, going round the circle calling players' names until everyone in the circle has had their name chanted.

Suggestion

The noise level of this activity can be adjusted by instructing players to stamp and chant quietly. The keeping of the rhythm can be supported with a drum.

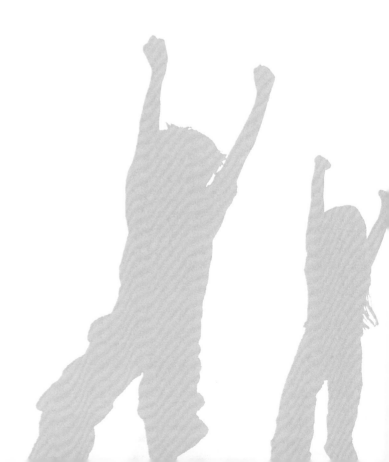

Circle of Names

This is a group gelling activity with a simple repeated structure.

Organisation of players

Players stand in a circle and take it in turns to go into the middle.

Playing the game

1   One player starts by going into the middle of the circle.

2   He says his name and another word beginning with the initial letter or initial sound of his name, for example, 'Jumping Jack', 'Smiling Sarah' or 'Clever Kyle'. The player also makes a gesture.

3   Everyone in the circle repeats the name, word and gesture back to the player.

4   He then stands back in the circle and another player goes into the middle, giving their name, word and gesture.

5   Everyone in the circle takes a turn in the middle.

6   The first player goes back into the middle of the circle.

7   He says nothing while the players in the circle recall his name, word and gesture and repeat these to him.

8   He then rejoins the circle.

9   Following the same sequence of players, each child goes back into the middle to have their name, word and gesture repeated to them.

Suggestion

If a child has difficulty thinking of a word or gesture, the group can help with this.

Rhythmic Hey-ho

In this game, the group take turns in a call and response sequence.

Organisation of players

Players stand in a circle, sideways on and all facing the same way. One player is the caller.

Playing the game

1   The game begins with players establishing a rhythmic back and forth movement, swinging their arms into and out of the circle as if they are brushing with an imaginary sweeping brush. Players should try and go in and out of the circle together.

2   Once the rhythm has been established, the caller calls out to the other players in a singsong way, 'Hey-ho'.

3   The other players in the circle echo this back together, calling out 'Hey-hey-hey-ho', maintaining their rhythmic movement as they do so.

4   The caller repeats this call and response sequence a few times.

5   Another player takes on the role of caller.

Suggestion

Some groups might find it easier to use a piece of equipment such as a parachute to achieve the same effect. The group stand in a circle holding the sides of the parachute. It is lifted up in the air and the caller calls, 'Hey-ho' to the group. As it falls and reveals the players to each other, they call back, 'Hey-hey-hey-ho'. In this way, the lifting and falling of the parachute creates a steady rhythm. Instead of 'hey-ho', children's names can be called.

Jack in the Box

This is a game for children to play in groups of five or six.

Organisation of players

All the players except one stand in a line facing forward. One player stands a little apart, facing the player who is at the front of the line. The player is holding a soft ball or a beanbag.

Playing the game

1   The player throws the ball to the first player in the line.

2   This player throws the ball back and crouches down, revealing the player who is standing behind her.

3   The player facing the group then throws the ball to this player, who throws it back and crouches down.

4   Players take it in turns to catch the ball and crouch down, following the sequence of the line.

Suggestion

This is a game to practise several times until players achieve a satisfying rhythm to the throwing and crouching down. Children who are better at catching and throwing should stand near the back of the line since they have to throw the ball over a greater distance.

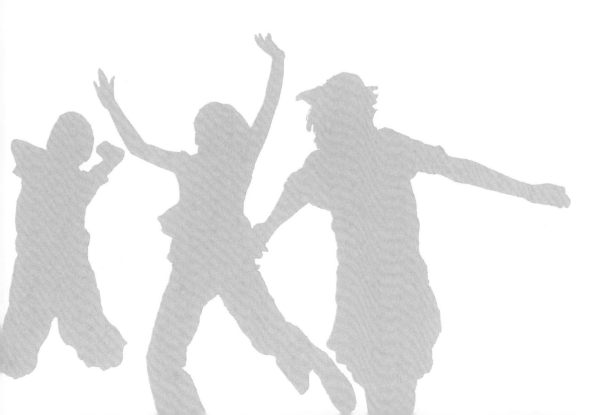

Leapfrog

This is a cooperative game with the rhythm of leaping and crouching down.

Organisation of players

Mark a starting line and a finishing line on the ground. Leave enough space between the start and finish for all the players to crouch down a short distance apart. Players line up behind the starting line.

Playing the game

1   The first player crouches down at the starting line.

2   The second player leaps over her and crouches down where he lands.

3   The third player then leaps over these two players in turn and crouches down.

4   Players continue to do this, leaping and crouching over the other players.

5   The final player in the line jumps over all the other jumping players and should cross the finishing line.

Suggestion

Alternatively, this game can be played in pairs with partners taking turns to crouch and leap over. The game is easier if players crouch down low so that others only need to jump over them. It is more difficult if players only bend over, so that other players have to vault over them.

Think About!

Acceptance

Keeping a steady rhythm in play is hard for many children with autism, who often require more time to respond and may have difficulty with the motor elements of a game. However, the sense of achieving a satisfying rhythm within a game depends on more than one individual. The social impairment of autism is to some extent a shared impairment, where the sense of success or failure in interaction involves more than one person. Slight variation in the rhythm of play is something that is either accepted by other children, or not. This depends largely on the culture of acceptance within the group, the degree of competition that exists and the skill of individual children to incorporate rhythmic missteps into the general play. Children should be praised for waiting patiently while another player takes their turn and for working together as a group rather than for the achievement of the rhythm itself.

Children think about:

When I am playing with other children, I sometimes have to wait my turn to start playing.

I start playing:

• when someone says, 'Ready, steady, go'

• when the person next to me has finished their turn

• by trying to keep to a rhythm

Ticking Clock

Ideally, this game should be played by 13 players, although any number will do.

Organisation of players

Twelve players stand in a circle, standing at an equal distance about a metre apart. One player in the circle holds a ball. The remaining player stands outside the circle, next to the player who is holding the ball.

Playing the game

1   The player with the ball throws it to the next player. At the same time, the player on the outside of the group starts to run round the circle.

2   The ball continues to be thrown around the circle, each player throwing it to his immediate neighbour.

3   The player on the outside of the circle runs all the way round. When she completes the circle, the player who has the ball at the time keeps hold of it.

4   The number of 'ticks of the clock' – the number of times the ball has been thrown – is counted to see how fast the player ran.

5   Another player takes the role of runner and the game is repeated.

6   By the end of the game, each player should have a score for how many ticks of the clock it took them to run round the circle.

Suggestion

The game can be played with any number of players, as long as they can create a big enough circle to run round without leaving too much distance between players.

High and Low Claps

In this game players must try to achieve an up and down rhythmic movement.

Organisation of players

Players stand in a circle.

Playing the game

1   One player starts by turning to another. They clap together, holding their hands high up above their heads or bending down and clapping low by their feet. Whether the first clap is high or low is determined by the starting player.

2   The second player then turns to his neighbour on the other side. They clap together, doing a clap that is the opposite of the previous clap. If the first clap was high, then the second should be low.

3   The clap is passed round the circle in this way, alternating between high and low claps, until it returns to the first player.

4   Another player starts the game again.

Suggestion

It is hard to get this game right the first time, but with practice groups can become adept at clapping high and low.

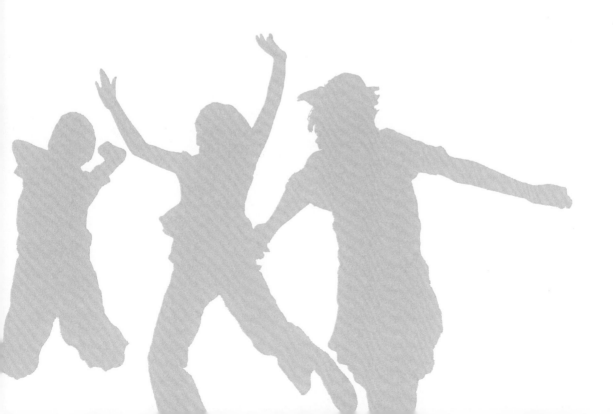

Blanket Tennis

In this game, using a blanket helps the group to coordinate their actions.

Organisation of players

The group divides into two. Each group has a blanket. There is one soft ball between the two groups.

Playing the game

1   In their groups, players take hold of the blanket and stretch it out until it is tight.

2   One group starts by placing the ball in the middle of their blanket.

3   They toss the ball in the air a few times to build up momentum.

4   They then try to toss the ball over into the blanket of the second group.

5   The second group try to catch the ball.

6   They then do the same, build up momentum and toss the ball across.

7   The two groups keep up this blanket tennis for as many turns as they can manage.

Suggestion

To make the game more difficult, groups must stand on either side of a net or another obstacle. The ball must be passed over the net before being caught by the other side.

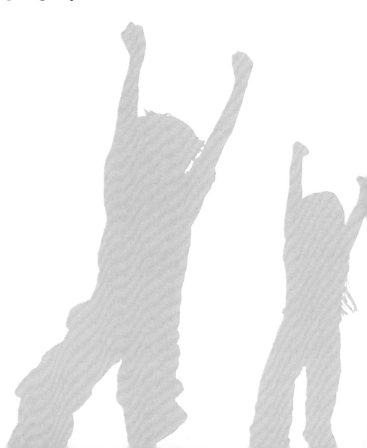

Rhythm Shoes

This is a game where a group is challenged to keep to a rhythm.

Organisation of players

Players sit in a circle. Each player puts one of their shoes on the floor in front of them.

Playing the game

1   A simple rhythm is established for the group to follow. This may be one player using a drum, one player clapping or the group themselves calling a rhythm, such as 'Tick-tock, tick-tock'.

2   In time with the rhythm, players pass the shoes around the circle. For example, the play may go 'Tick' (pass a shoe), 'Tock' (pass a shoe) and so on.

3   The object of the game is for the shoes to be passed round with no player having two shoes in front of him at any time.

4   If the group lose the rhythm, they can begin again.

Suggestion

Some children with autism do not like their possessions being touched by other people. If players do not want to use their shoes, any other object can be used such as beanbags or books.

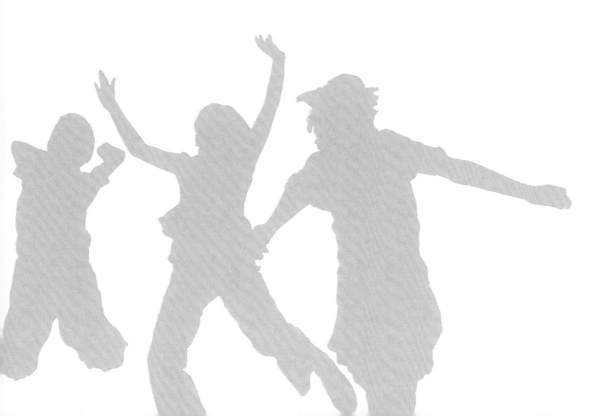

Two Canes

This game can be played at a rhythmic pace that suits the players.

Organisation of players

Two players stand holding two long canes horizontally between them, one cane in each hand.

Playing the game

1   The two players with the canes set up a rhythm by raising one cane as they lower the other. The rise and fall of the canes should follow a slow and steady 'tick-tock' rhythm.

2   The other players stand close by.

3   Players take turns to approach the canes. They must try to synchronise their movements with the canes, walking through them without touching them, stepping over one and going under the other.

4   The whole group of players can try to establish a rhythm of walking through the canes so that there is a steady and continuous stream of children going through.

Suggestion

The players holding the canes should be encouraged to make a rhythm that suits the other players and is neither too fast nor too slow.

Cooperation

2 Games of togetherness

Like rhythmic games, games of togetherness provide a clear interactional sequence within the play, but with much greater emphasis on the experience of shared feeling between players. These games promote the idea that, in playing together, players can experience an emotional connection between them. For this purpose, the games use experiences such as being copied by another player, working together as a group to create a physical effect in a game and listening out for another player with eyes closed. Trust is an important element in many of these games, adding a further emotional dimension for players.

Key terms

following, moving at the same time, learning to trust

Progression of skills

• copy one other player

• work together to produce an effect

• be playful in a coordinated way

• show trust in other players.

Follow the Leader

This well-known game requires children to copy the player in front of them.

Organisation of players

One player is the leader. All the other players line up behind him.

Playing the game

1 The leader sets off on a route of his own choosing with all the players following him.

2 He performs any actions that he can think of, for example, running in a zigzag, jumping a number of times, going under a wall, hopping, walking along a bench.

3 The players following him must copy these actions as accurately as possible.

4 After a while, a new leader is chosen and the game begins again.

5 Leaders can choose to perform actions of their own or actions that have already been used.

Suggestion

Another way of playing this game is in a circle. One player is the leader and all the other players must copy his movements, gestures, sounds and facial expressions while staying in the circle.

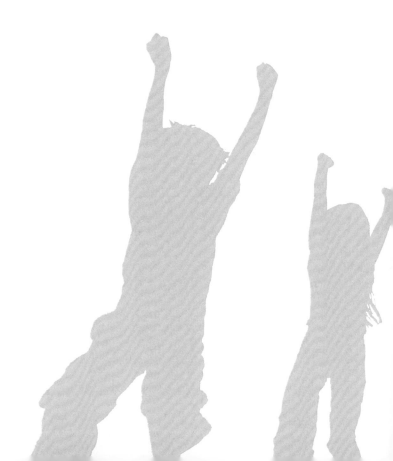

Mirror

Players mirror each other's movements in pairs.

Organisation of players

Players divide into two lines and stand facing each other, each player lined up with a partner in the opposite line. One line, line B, is the 'mirror'.

Playing the game

1   The players in line A begin to make their own individual movements. They can move their arms, legs, face, hands and body, but must stay roughly in the line.

2   The players in line B begin to copy the movements of their partner in line A.

3   Players should not move too quickly to make sure that their partner in line B can keep up with their movements.

4   Players mirror each other in this way for a short time and then swap roles.

Suggestion

Copying the movements of another person requires some skill and may be difficult for some children. If this is the case, it is not necessary for children to swap the roles of mover and mirror.

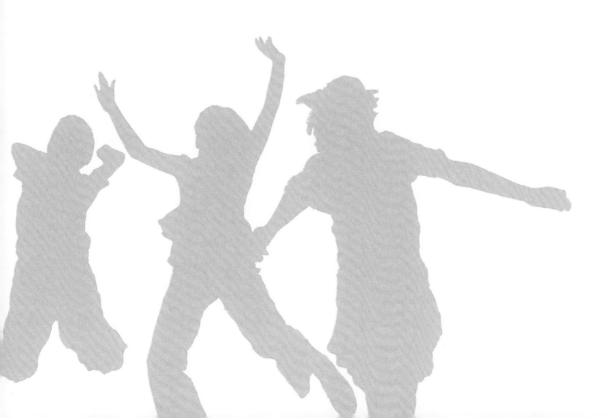

Think About!

Building trust

Trust is not something that is just there at the beginning of a relationship or an interaction, but must be earned over time. Trust is earned through repeated experiences of positive and reliable interaction, doing something again and again in a predictable way while taking care of others and having fun together. Games are an ideal way of developing a sense of trust among players. Children like to play the same games over and over again. Moreover, games themselves often involve a ritual, an act that is performed in a preordained way and repeated by the players. Many games, too, require players to work together in a cooperative way, coordinating their movements, looking out for each other and protecting other players' interests. Children should be praised for playing safely with one another and challenged to do this even when playing more physically exertive games.

Children think about:

Playing safely with others means:

S – Stick to the same way of doing something

A – Always think of others

F – Feet, hands and knees – keep them in check

E – Everyone enjoys themselves

Walking Backwards

This game requires children to work together in pairs.

Organisation of players

Players are in pairs; one player is the leader and the other the follower.

Playing the game

1 The player who is following closes her eyes and stands with their back to their partner. He faces the follower, standing close to her.

2 The leader starts to walk slowly backwards. As he walks he makes a humming sound, not too loud but loud enough for his partner to hear.

3 The player who is following, still with eyes closed, tries to follow her partner wherever he goes, walking backwards.

4 After a while, the leader stops humming and stops walking. The follower must then stop too, trying not to bump into him.

Suggestion

Make sure partners have enough space to move around in, without bumping into other pairs. Leaders should take care of their partner, trying to build a situation of trust.

Hand Towers

This is a game of coordinated action.

Organisation of players

Players stand in a tight circle, turned sideways on and all facing in the same direction.

Playing the game

1 Players extend one arm into the middle of the circle. All players should use the same arm (right or left depending on which way they are facing in the circle). They must stand sufficiently close to one another for their hands to meet in the middle.

2 Players form a hand tower by placing their hand on top of, but not touching, that of another player.

3 The tower should be a long line of hands that are in line with each other but not touching.

4 Once the tower is formed, players can dismantle it. They do this by the player with the top hand slowly lifting it up and away in a smooth arc.

5 Players follow, taking turns in order to swing their hand away from the tower. The effect should be of hands slowly fanning away from the tower, rather than all being removed at once.

Suggestion

As players become adept at forming and dismantling hand towers, they can perform the actions in a continuous sequence. As the last player swings his hand away, the player whose hand was at the top starts a new tower by putting her hand into that bottom position.

Automatic Doors

In this game players must synchronise their movements to give an experience of coordinated group action.

Organisation of players

All players except one stand facing forward a little distance apart in two parallel lines. They hold out one arm, touching fingers lightly with the player who is standing next to them. The one remaining player stands at the end of the two lines of players.

Playing the game

1 Holding arms out, palms together, the player moves slowly towards the line of arms.

2 As the player approaches, the arms of the first two players in the line open as the players move their arms sideways. The effect should be of automatic doors opening at the approach of someone walking towards them.

3 The arms of the remaining players open in this way in a coordinated fashion, so that they open as the player approaches them.

4 When the players has gone through the line of arms, another player takes his place and the game begins again.

Suggestion

It is important that this game is played slowly to give players the chance to coordinate their arm movements. The more the game is played, the better children get at coordinating their movements.

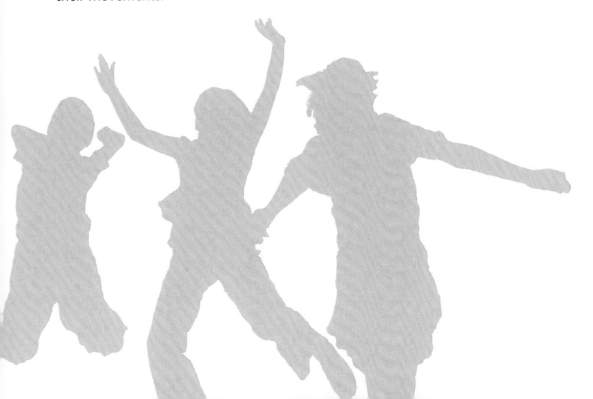

Lion Listening

In this game one player must listen carefully for other players' movements.

Organisation of players

One player volunteers to be the lion. She sits in the centre of the players, who sit higgledy-piggledy in the play space. An object is placed next to the lion.

Playing the game

1 The player who is the lion is blindfolded or closes their eyes.

2 Players take it in turns to slowly approach the lion. They may stand up and walk towards the lion or crawl along the floor.

3 The player who is the lion listens for the movement of a player. When she hears someone she points at him.

4 If the lion points accurately at a player, he must return to where he was sitting. If not, the player can continue approaching the lion.

5 When a player reaches the object, the lion takes off her blindfold and swaps places with the player.

Suggestion

As a way of making the game more difficult, players must take the object, which is placed on something, such as a plastic bag, that will make a noise when it is lifted.

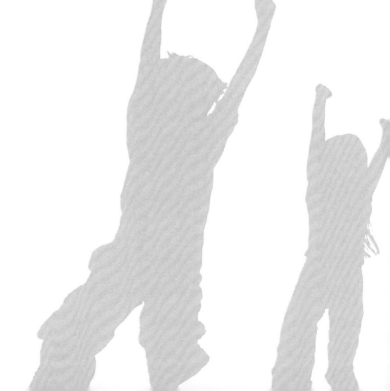

Grandma's Glasses

This is a traditional game that sets up an exciting connection between two players.

Organisation of players

One player is Grandma and sits on a chair pretending to be asleep. She should have a pair of glasses in her pocket, sticking out slightly, or resting on her lap. The other players stand a short distance away from her.

Playing the game

1   When it is clear that Grandma is asleep, players take it in turns to approach her, moving as quietly as possible.

2   If Grandma wakes up and sees a player moving, she sends him back to the line of other players. However, if the player freezes before Grandma opens her eyes, she must go back to sleep.

3   When a player reaches Grandma, he must try to take her glasses out of her pocket without waking her up.

Suggestion

This game is helped if the player who is Grandma does not wake up too often and allows other players to get close to her. Sometimes it is better to have an adult or an older child play Grandma in the game, the other children simply approaching her.

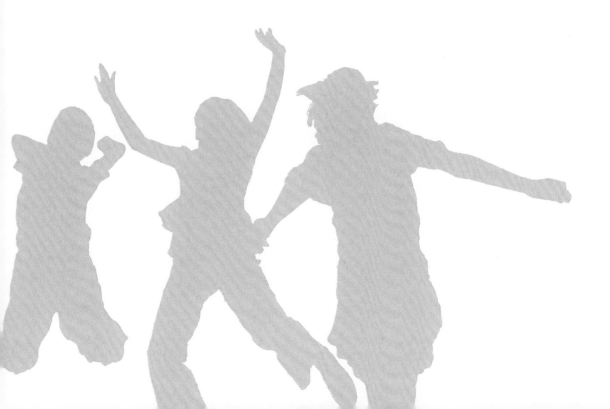

Cat and Mouse Circles

This is an exciting game in which players move together to protect one member of the circle.

Organisation of players

All the players except one stand in a circle holding hands. This player, the cat, stands outside the circle. One player in the circle is chosen or volunteers to be the mouse.

Playing the game

1   The cat must try to tag the mouse.

2   Remaining in the circle and holding hands, the mouse must try to escape from the cat by moving away from him.

3   The whole circle works together to protect the mouse from the cat, circling away from the cat's approaches.

Suggestion

Children may need the strict instruction not to let go of hands or move too far away from the cat. The area in which the circle turns can be marked out in chalk.

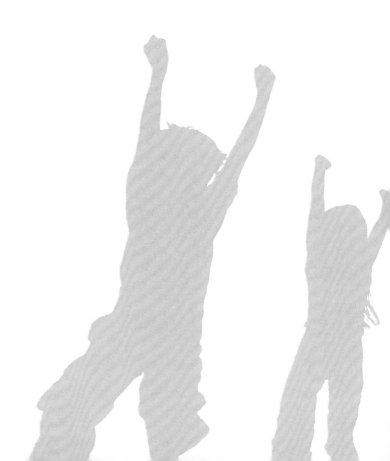

Falling Backwards

This is a game of trust played as a whole group.

Organisation of players

A play area is clearly designated which players freely walk round.

Playing the game

1   Any player can decide to fall backwards at any point.

2   As he is about to fall, he calls out 'Falling!' and slowly begins to fall backwards.

3   At this signal, other nearby players rush to catch the player who is falling.

4   As soon as the person is caught safely, the game can begin again.

Suggestion

If playing the game in this way is too difficult for a group, falling backwards can be done without walking around the space. Players can simply take it in turns to fall backwards with a line of players standing behind to catch them.

Instead of players calling out 'Falling', a caller can be used for this, watching out for players who are beginning to fall. Children may also need instruction in how to fall backwards slowly, giving others enough time to catch them, and in how to catch someone safely.

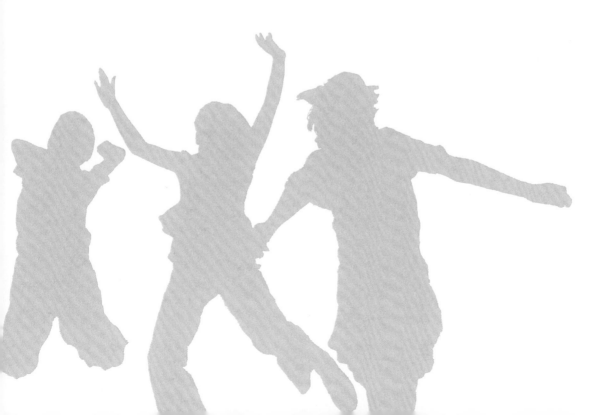

Group Lifts

This game can give a powerful experience of trust within a group.

Organisation of players

One volunteer lies on the floor or on a bench. The remaining players stand around him.
A sponge mat may be placed under the player who is lifted.

Playing the game

1   Players space themselves equally around the player who is to be lifted and put their hands a little way underneath him.

2   One player counts down to the lift, 'One, two, three, lift!'

3   Working together, players lift up the player who is lying down.

4   The player is initially lifted waist high.

5   A prearranged signal, such as a nod, can be used by the player to indicate that he wants to go higher.

Suggestion

This is a skilful game that requires the group to lift safely in a coordinated way. It also depends on the player who is being lifted to trust the group and allow himself to be lifted. It is not a game that all children will enjoy, though some will like it immensely. It is important that children volunteer to be lifted.

Cooperation

3 Looking and finding games

The earliest games involve looking for someone who is hiding and taking pleasure in finding them. Peekaboo is perhaps the first game that infants play and is made up of just these elements: looking for someone who is hiding and who knows they are being looked for, the excitement that this knowledge brings and the final dramatic act of being found. Playing such games is an immensely emotional experience that is related to the attachment behaviours of children and their parents.

There is a developmental progression to such games, from 'When I shut my eyes I can't be seen' to 'When I shut my eyes other people disappear'. Gradually, children learn to consider the other person's point of view and realise that they themselves must be hidden. Children with autism demonstrate attachment behaviour, but typically show confusion when playing hiding games. They need to learn what is required of them by playing less sophisticated versions.

The games in this section build up this understanding while focusing on the important emotional aspect of taking pleasure in finding someone. The first two games focus on finding without any special kind of seeking. The focus here is on greeting someone who has been found. The next three games involve keeping someone in mind, thinking about them even when they cannot be seen. The final five games focus on hunting as a skill. Three games practise the skill of looking for clues in the environment, scanning and noticing small details. The final two games, which include Hide-and-Seek itself, practise exploring the play space in a systematic way.

Key terms
greeting with pleasure, holding someone in mind, the play area

Progression of skills
• greet with pleasure

• hold another person in mind

• the play area – look for clues

• the play area – use the space systematically.

Boo!

This game is about finding places to hide that are fun and greeting players who have been hiding.

Organisation of players

Players walk around the environment looking for good places to hide themselves. These could be behind curtains, under the stairs, in a cupboard, and so on.

Playing the game

1   Players try out different hiding places, hiding themselves and then jumping out to reveal themselves.

2   Players take turns to try out the hiding place and reveal themselves in a dramatic way.

3   Other players are encouraged to greet the hiding player when she is revealed. They can say, 'Hello ___!' or applaud when she is seen.

Suggestion

Instead of players hiding themselves, toys can be used to give the same experience. Toys that can be hidden and then automatically pop up or jump out are ideal. Have fun with the surprise and pleasure that these toys give.

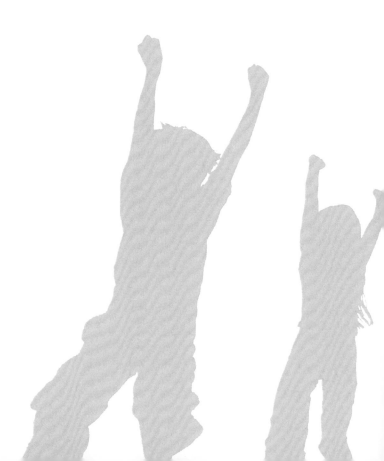

Come Out, Come Out, Wherever You Are

This is a simple seeking game in which players are not expected to be expert at hiding themselves. There is no real hunting element, only seeing and naming players.

Organisation of players

One player is chosen to be the seeker while the other players find a hiding space.

Playing the game

1   The seeker goes out of the room or covers her eyes.

2   Players are told to hide themselves somewhere and try to stay quiet.

3   The seeker stands in a prominent position and looks around the space, looking for players.

4   When she sees one, she calls out to them 'I can see ___', naming the player.

5   That player stands up. Players greet each other by saying 'Hello' or smiling. The player remains standing in their place until the game is finished.

6   All players are called out in this way. If a player cannot be seen, they are asked to make a noise or show a limb to reveal their whereabouts.

Suggestion

This game benefits from players not hiding themselves properly and is a good antecedent to more sophisticated hiding games. It works well in a small space where players can more easily be seen and heard. Players can reveal themselves in a dramatic or funny way, popping up from their hiding place or jumping out.

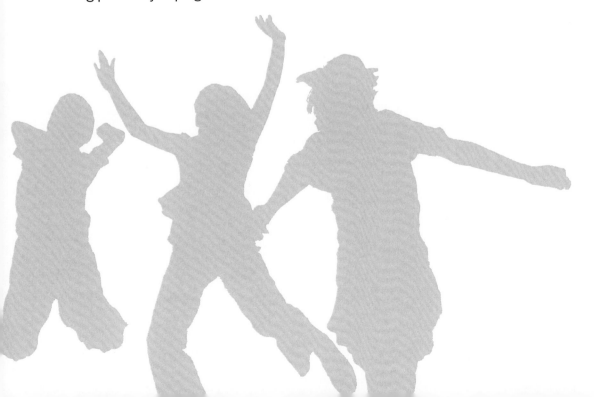

Hiding Under the Blanket

The beauty of this game is that the player who is hiding is still clearly in view, but their identity is unknown.

Organisation of players

Players lie higgledy-piggledy on the ground face down, instructed not to look.

Playing the game

1   One player is covered with a thick blanket so that no part of their body can be seen.

2   Players are told to stand up and make a circle round the hidden player.

3   The outline of the player who is hiding is visible, but they cannot be seen and other players must guess who is hiding under the blanket.

4   When a player guesses correctly, the player under the blanket is revealed.

5   The game begins again.

Suggestion

In this game, players must think about who is missing in their group by looking to see who is standing in the circle. It works better with slightly larger groups.

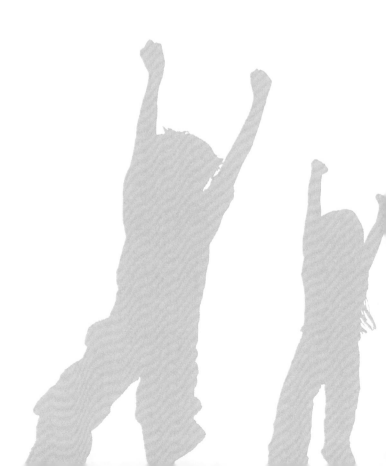

Whose Face?

This is a funny guessing game that plays with the idea of not being able to see someone you know is there.

Organisation of players

Players sit in a line on chairs or on the floor.

Playing the game

1   One player volunteers to be blindfold and sits facing the group.

2   Another player silently volunteers to have her face felt and stands in front of the player who is blindfolded.

3   The blindfolded player feels her face.

4   The player whose face has been felt sits back in her place.

5   The player removes his blindfold and guesses whose face he has just felt.

Suggestion

An alternative way to play Whose face? is as a 'Freeze' game. One player is blindfolded and stands in the middle of the group. Players walk around until a caller says, 'Freeze!' The blindfolded player now starts to move, searching around for a player whose face she feels and identifies.

Check whether players are happy to be blindfold. Most children will be happy with the idea, but some may not. Point out the aspects of someone's appearance that reveal their identity: their long hair, for example, or smiling face.

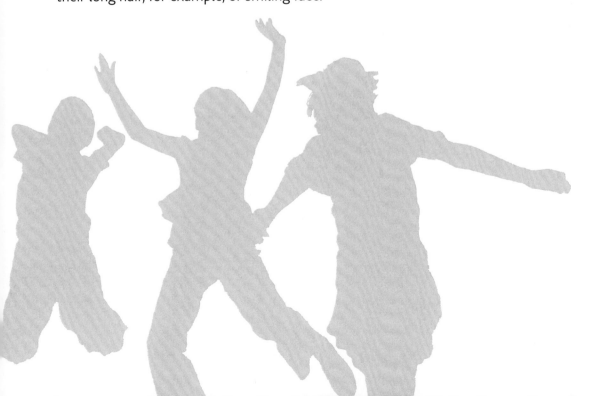

Who Is It?

This game plays with the idea that someone knows something that you do not, but that you can find out by asking them questions.

Organisation of players

The players sit in a row.

Playing the game

1 One player volunteers and sits with her back to the group.

2 Another player volunteers to describe a third player.

3 A third player is silently chosen to be described.

4 The describer gives a description of this player, giving details of his appearance, personality or special interests.

5 The player with her back to the group must guess the identity of the player being described.

6 When she guesses correctly, she turns round to verify the description.

Suggestion

Encourage the idea of creating mental pictures of other people. Talk about the fact that you can see people in your mind even when you cannot see them in reality.

Think About!

Mapping out the play area

The area in which children play a game is an important but largely abstract concept. Knowing where to play and staying within boundaries is something with which many children have trouble. Games differ in terms of the use and amount of area needed for the play. Children play games in different places too, needing to re-establish boundaries each time. Hunting games can be particularly problematic in terms of the play area, with children searching far and wide for someone or something. When playing these next games, be sure to clearly point out the physical boundaries of a game before beginning to play it.

Fortunately there are a number of ways children traditionally use to help them keep the play space in mind. Typically they use natural boundaries to demarcate where players can and cannot go. Walls, corners of buildings, trees and lines of the playground are all good visual ways of marking out play boundaries. Natural boundaries can be visually enhanced with the use of other markers. Jumpers and coats can be used for this purpose, as well as more colourful items such as flags or marker cones. Some children may require more autism-specific strategies, with 'start' and 'finish' symbols or green and red markers to indicate 'go' and 'stop' placed in strategic positions.

Children think about:

I play games with my friends. Sometimes we play indoors and sometimes we play outside. When we play a game I should try to stay within a certain area. This is known as the area we play in or play area.

The area we play in is not always the same. Sometimes it might be the playground, sometimes it might be only part of the playground. When I start playing a game I can ask about the area we are playing in for this game. I can ask where we can run to, how far we can go and where we should not go.

Huckle, Buckle, Beanstalk

This game practises the skill of scanning the play area to look for clues without actually physically moving through the space to hunt.

Organisation of players

The game can be played outside, but is probably better played indoors. Players must hunt with their eyes only – no moving around the space is allowed.

Playing the game

1   One player holds up an object for the other players to see.

2   Players close their eyes or go out of the room while the first player hides the object.

3   The object should not be completely hidden: a small part remains in view. The degree to which it can be seen should be determined by the skilfulness of the players who will be looking for it.

4   Players open their eyes or return to the room. They are told where to stand and in which area they must look for the object.

5   Players begin scanning the designated area for the object.

6   When a player spots the object, he says 'Huckle, buckle, beanstalk' and sits down. He should avoid pointing out the whereabouts of the object to the other players.

7   The game ends when all players have spotted the object or the set time for the game has run out.

Suggestion

Some children find scanning the environment difficult and may find it hard to spot the object. It is possible to play the game one-on-one, with one player hiding the object and only one player at a time looking for it. This allows players to find their own pace in the game.

Photo Hunt

This is a wonderful game for learning to decode clues. The difficulty of the clues can be adjusted according to the skill of the players.

Organisation of players

The game works well outside in a large hunting area, though can be played indoors. Be clear about the boundaries of the hunt. Clues must be in place before the game begins and may be best set by an adult.

Playing the game

1   To set up the game, one player or an adult plants a series of clues. Clues take the form of a photograph of the object for which the players must search. Clues should be set in as creative a way as possible. For more experienced players, photos may be of only a detail of that object.

2   Each clue contains sufficient information to lead players to the next clue in a sequence, the final clue leading to some sort of treasure.

3   Players are given the first clue and then set off to look for that object.

4   It is possible to organise players into small teams with the treasure at the end held by an adult outside the game.

Suggestion

A nice alternative to this game is to incorporate the special interests of a child with autism. Objects can be chosen that relate to this, for example, a book about the subject or a small toy of the subject. Alternatively, pieces of a jigsaw puzzle can be incorporated in the finding of objects. Each piece should go to making up the jigsaw so that the final clue yields not only some treasure but the last piece of the jigsaw puzzle.

Hide the Ball

This is a good exercise in cooperation since players must work together to keep a hunter from tracking down a hidden ball.

Organisation of players

Players sit or stand in a tight circle, with no spaces between them and with their hands behind their backs. The larger the number of players in the circle the better.

Playing the game

1 One player is chosen or volunteers to sit in the centre of the circle. He closes his eyes and counts to ten.

2 A ball is passed from one player in the circle to the next, passing it behind their backs.

3 When the player in the middle reaches ten, the players stop passing the ball. The player who has the ball must hide it as best she can.

4 The player in the middle tries to work out who has the ball by looking carefully around the circle.

5 He calls out the name of a player he suspects has the ball, who must then show her hands.

6 If he has guessed correctly, they swap places; if not, he must count again.

Suggestion

This game can be made easier or more difficult by altering the size of the ball. Smaller balls are easier to conceal, but larger balls require more skill on the part of the player who is hiding it – to hide the ball and keep a straight face. Be sure to point out to the group what type of clues they are looking for and what makes someone look suspicious.

Cold, Hot and Boiling

This is a difficult game which equates the nearness of the hunter to the hidden object with the concept of 'warming up' and increasing distance with 'growing colder'.

Organisation of players

An object is hidden and one player hunts for it. Before the hunting begins, establish clear boundaries for the hunting area. Specify which area signifies 'cold', which area 'hot' and which area 'boiling'.

Playing the game

1   One player is sent out of the room or out of sight while the other players hide an object.

2   The player returns and is given the parameters in which to hunt. He begins to search for the object.

3   As he searches, the other players provide clues by calling out 'You're getting warmer' when he moves into that part of the play space, 'You're getting colder' when he moves out of the hunting space, and 'You're boiling!' when he is close to the object.

4   When the player finds the object, the game begins again using another hiding space with new 'cold', 'hot' and 'boiling' boundaries.

Suggestion

As a way of simplifying the game, the boundaries for 'cold', 'hot' and 'boiling' can remain the same for each turn, marked out with blue, orange and red coloured markers.

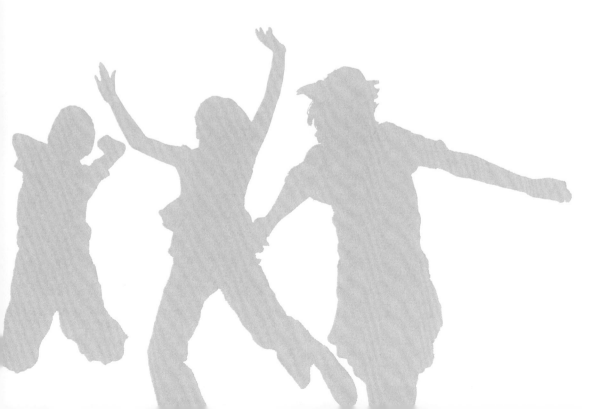

Hide-and-Seek

Hide-and-seek is a very old game that takes many different forms. Here it is played as a seeking game without the added sophistication of a chase home.

Organisation of players

One player is 'It' and other players hide. The boundaries for where hiding can take place are clearly described to all the players before the game begins.

Playing the game

1 The player who is 'It' closes his eyes and counts to 50 while the other players find hiding places.

2 When the player has finished counting, he shouts out, 'Ready or not, here I come!' and begins looking for hidden players.

3 The player who is hunting should be encouraged to move through the whole area of the playing space, being reminded where he has not yet been.

4 When a player is found, the hunter calls out, 'I spy ___ (the player's name) behind the cupboard!' (giving the whereabouts of hider).

Suggestion

Some children may require support for this game, beyond having the extent of the play area defined. For some, it may be necessary to explain what makes a good hiding place or even to point out good places to hide. Others may need a partner with whom to hide or hunt.

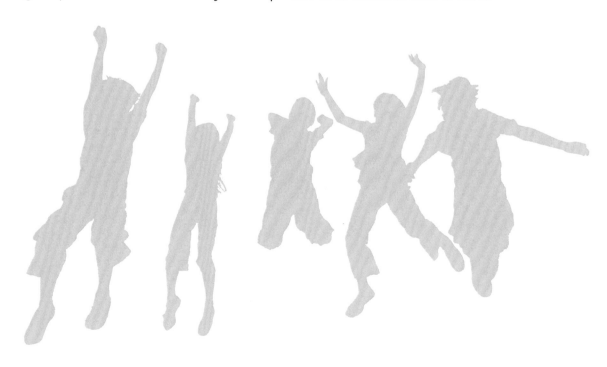

Self-regulation

Self-regulation refers to the ability we have to control our attention, our level of arousal and our actions. Exercising this kind of control means being able to organise our attention by cutting out peripheral stimuli, cope with excited feelings, exert ourselves physically and inhibit physical and mental impulses. Our ability to do these things is based in the body but relates strongly to our mental processes as well. It could be said, in fact, that the body is part of the mind. The control of our attention, feelings and actions is not something of which we are always fully conscious, yet is evidence of the way our thought processes work. Rather than a conscious taking in of and thinking about experience as it happens to us, our responses are much more instantaneous and body-based.

Self-regulation is part of the disorder of autism and the reason why people with autism sometimes respond to their environment differently. Children with autism can become fixated on something in the environment, unable to switch their attention from it. Equally, they may have difficulty controlling their attention on something, may become over-stimulated and may have to withdraw completely in order to switch off their attention.

The games listed here are designed to help children regulate their physical responses through improved self-awareness and bodily control. They are aimed at developing body awareness by using games that involve strength and at developing attention by encouraging children to be more consciously aware of their perceptions. They should also help children cope more effectively with the feeling of excitement in games.

It is important to remember that all children need sensitive and gentle support when learning to self-regulate. As babies, all children require a carer who provides positive encouragement for their efforts, allowing them to turn away or withdraw completely when they become too uncomfortable or aroused. In playing the following games, be aware that children need positive experiences of physical effort and lots of praise. Point out when a child demonstrates he has coped with something, regulated his feelings or exerted himself physically, explaining what he has done and why it is something good.

Self-regulation

4 Games of exertion

Games of exertion require players to use their physical strength with or against other players. All the games described here involve pushing, pulling and gripping movements in a controlled, focused and determined way. The aim of the games is to use strength, but not mindlessly.

Importantly, games of exertion develop proprioceptive awareness. Proprioception is our sensory system that provides feedback from inside the body and gives us an internal awareness of our bodily self. Proprioceptive activity relates to the development of a sense of self and a sense of others. It gives rise to self-control and the ability to act in a coordinated fashion with others, contributing to a sense of mastery and self-confidence.

For children with autism, motor control and muscular strength are often areas of difficulty. It is unclear what the relation of motor development is to that of social understanding, but motor difficulty does impact adversely on our sense of ourselves, of others and of the environment, with probable repercussions for social development. The games in this section focus on different aspects of physical exertion, from simple gripping activities to a more determined and controlled use of pushing, pulling and body strength.

Key terms
being strong, persevering, controlling strength, confidence

Progression of skills
• exert strength in a purposeful way

• persevere in physical exertion

• control strength and be mindful of other players.

Parcels

This game requires players to keep a tight control of themselves physically by maintaining a firm grip. It gives an actual bodily experience of self-control and provides a good starting point for this section of games.

Organisation of players

Players take turns to curl up to make a parcel, hugging their knees with a good grip. An adult – and possibly an assistant or older children – tests the strength of each player by gently trying to unfold them.

Playing the game

1   The adult 'tests' a player's strength by gently pulling on his limbs. The aim is not to open the parcel, but to encourage the player to resist the pulling.

2   Players come forward to take turns to make parcels. Other children watch and enjoy the game.

3   Children should be praised for working hard in the pose. They should be described as 'strong' or 'determined'.

4   For a child who is able to maintain a strong grip, the adult can lift him up, holding him around the waist and gently swinging him.

5   The adult can take a turn to curl up. Several children at a time can try to uncurl her.

Suggestion

Children need to be fairly light to be lifted. However, anyone, whatever their size, can be tested by others pulling on their arms and legs to try to uncurl them. There should be positive reinforcement throughout for the need to pull *gently*.

See-Saw

The aim of this game is to achieve a coordinated rhythm through careful partnership work.

Organisation of players

Players sit on the floor in pairs, facing each other and holding each other's forearms (not hands). Partners should establish a good grip. Feet should be flat on the floor, toe to toe with the partner, and knees bent.

Playing the game

1   Players decide who will rise up first. The pair brace themselves, getting ready to pull.

2   One partner rises, pulled up by the other.

3   When he reaches standing, he goes down again slowly. As he does so, his partner begins to rise.

4   Partners should try to achieve a rhythm to their movement, moving up and down smoothly and continuously as if they were playing on a real see-saw.

5   A variation is for both partners to achieve a standing position by pulling themselves up together.

Suggestion

This game requires players to use the right amount of exertion to achieve a rhythm. They should pull neither too much nor too little. They must learn to regulate their exertion to the amount required by the weight of their partner. Swapping partners helps with this process of learning.

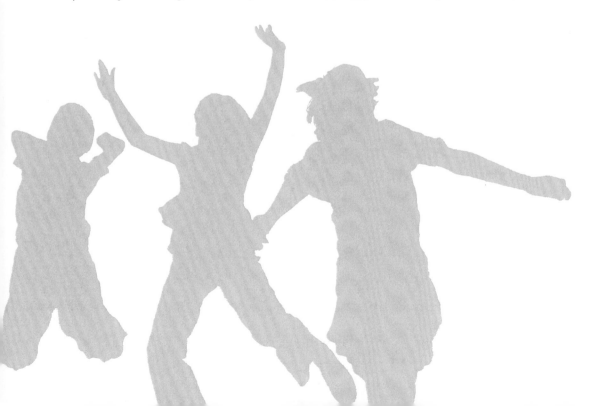

Balances

Children work in pairs to control their strength interactively and so achieve a balance.

Organisation of players

Players are put into pairs. Partners are roughly of equal size and build. Each pair of children sits back to back with their feet on the floor and knees bent.

Playing the game

1   In their pairs, children begin to gently push each other, slowly increasing the force of the push.

2   When they push with sufficient force, they should begin to rise up to standing.

3   Pushing should be 'interactive' so that a state of balance is achieved, with partners pushing with equal force.

4   They should hold the balance for a while and then begin to go down again, eventually coming to sit once more on the floor.

5   They can then try other positions to make balances: hands together and legs akimbo, shoulder to shoulder with legs away, feet together lying on their backs and with hands holding on the floor. The aim always is to achieve a balance and not push the partner over or away.

Suggestion

Some children have difficulty achieving this kind of interactive balance. If this is the case, place a piece of paper between the body parts being pushed together. The pair must then keep the paper in place by pushing against each other.

Grippy

This is a traditional game that is simple to play and highly enjoyable. It combines the two previous skills of maintaining a grip while using physical strength.

Organisation of players

Form groups of two or three players. One player holds a small object such as a coin or a button.

Playing the game

1   The player holding the small object makes her fist as tight as she can. When she is ready, she says 'Go!'

2   The others in the group try to force open her fist, pulling at her fingers.

3   Players take turns to hold the object and resist the others opening their fist.

Suggestion

As with many of the games in this section, the emphasis is on exerting yourself while being mindful of others. Key instructions are: gently, carefully, be aware of the other person's responses.

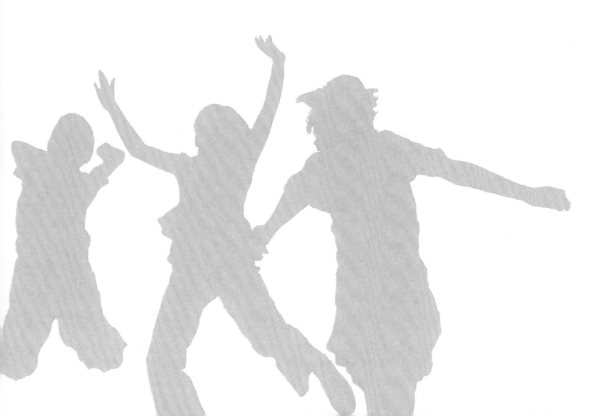

Roots

This game refers to the roots of a tree. Children should be asked to visualise the roots of a tree going deeply into the earth, ensuring it is strong and stable.

Organisation of players

Players form groups of three or four players. Children take turns to be moved by the others in the small group.

Playing the game

1 One player in each group volunteers to go first.

2 He is given some time to prepare himself, to become 'as immovable as a tree'.

3 When he is ready, he nods. The other children in his group take turns to try to push him over.

4 Another player volunteers to take a turn.

Suggestion

Children should be made aware that strength takes both a physical and a mental form.
In preparing themselves to resist the others, they should prepare themselves both physically and mentally. It does help if children visualise themselves as a strongly rooted tree with their strength going down into the floor like roots. A diagram of a tree with roots can be drawn to help them visualise this.

Shoulder-to-Shoulder

This game should be played in a slow and stately manner. Emphasis is less on 'being strong' and more on achieving a coordinated use of physical force.

Organisation of players

The group stand in a line with their backs to the wall.

Playing the game

1   Each player places her shoulders against the shoulders of her neighbours.

2   Children should try to 'glue' themselves to each other by pressing gently against each other's shoulders.

3   Once the whole line is glued together in this way, it moves forward as one line – no individual player should be ahead or behind the others and the line should not wobble or break.

4   The line moves across the room in a slow and stately fashion, proceeding to the opposite wall where the children can relax.

Suggestion

As an extension to this game, the group can go through an obstacle course. For example, they might sit on the floor together, turn a corner and sit on a row of chairs. The group can also try turning round together, re-gluing the line and retracing their route.

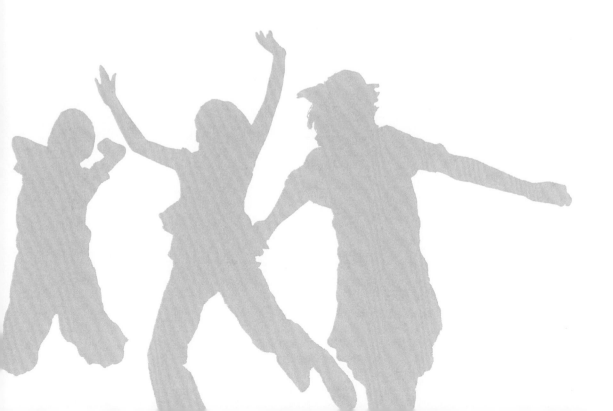

Jars of Honey

This is a traditional game which requires players to keep their grip, but has an added imaginative element with a ritualistic chant.

Organisation of players

One player is the shopkeeper, one a customer. The remaining children crouch down in a row holding their knees and pretending to be jars of honey.

Playing the game

1   The customer tells the shopkeeper that she would like to buy some honey.

2   She tastes the honey by touching each 'jar' on the head. As children are tapped on the head, the customer asks, 'Is it good or has it gone off?'

3   She selects one and, with the help of the shopkeeper, tests whether the jar of honey is intact. They take the crouching child under each arm and gently raise and lower him, swing and shake him, to see if he is any good.

4   The object of the game is to break the jar by forcing the child to let go of his knees. If this happens, the jar is rejected. The child must stand out of the line and the customer can continue.

5   If the jar holds, that is, the child manages to keep his grip, he becomes the new customer.

Suggestion

When the jar is tested, the customer and shopkeeper can together chant:

Is she rotten, is she sound

Is she worth a million pound?

Toss her up and toss her down

She is worth a million pound!

Statues

This game requires players to focus their strength in one part of their body, individual players deciding which part.

Organisation of players

With the group divided, half should become statues and half 'pullers'. The object of the game is for the pullers to pull the statues off balance by pulling on the part of the body that is sticking out.

Playing the game

1   Players who are statues find a space for themselves.

2   They become a statue, freezing in one position. One part of the body should be sticking out as something to pull: arm, elbow, leg, knee, foot, bottom or hip.

3   Pullers choose a statue or are assigned one. They stand in front of the statue and formally ask how statues want to be pulled, using the sentence 'Do you want to be pulled fast, slow, medium or with a twist?'

4   The statue chooses one and prepares for the pulling. The puller tries to pull the statue off balance by using only the part that is sticking out and the method of pulling chosen by the statue. The statue tries to resist.

5   Players reverse roles, the statues becoming pullers and vice versa.

Suggestion

An alternative way of playing the game is for statues to place a 'button' on themselves, indicating the spot at which they can be pushed. A badge can be pinned on to serve as a button to press. Children should experiment with the best places to resist another person's force.

Think About!

Aggression

Typically, aggression is associated with hostile and violent acts. However, the action referred to in the original root of the word is more benign in its definition, meaning 'to proceed' or 'to reach out'. This helps to remind us that aggression – the use of one's strength to obtain some means – can serve as a force for good. Using one's strength in a focused and persistent manner is an important skill in life and a powerful source of self-esteem.

Positive aggression is *controlled* aggression, where physical strength can be exerted but also reduced or stopped when necessary. It is important for children to understand that exertion has both a physical and a mental component; they must be *mindful* of their physical exertion and so have control over it. Children should have the experience of *thinking while acting*. They should be encouraged to combine mental focus with muscular strength. The instruction should be to push *carefully*, pull *gently*, to be aware of the other person, to act but to take care, and so on.

In this way, even games that are often deemed too aggressive to play – such as the following two games – can be played without harm and can give an experience of being able to both think and do.

Children think about:

I can use my muscles to be strong. I can push, pull and grip things. Sometimes when I play a game, I have to be strong.

When I play with my friends I must remember not to hurt them. I can enjoy myself and use my strength, but I must try to keep thinking about my friends in my mind.

Adder's Nest

This is a classic game of exertion that requires players to be physically persistent.

Organisation of players

The group is organised into circles of approximately 10 players holding hands. They circle an object that is in the middle of the circle, which could be a box, a jumper or something already built into the floor, such as a manhole cover.

Playing the game

1 The players circle the object.

2 One player declares that the object is poisonous, for example, 'This box is poisonous!'

3 At this signal, players try to force their neighbours to knock against the object in the circle, while avoiding it themselves. Players must not let go of hands but can push against their neighbours.

4 When a player touches the object, she must stand out of the circle.

Suggestion

Adder's Nest, like other traditional games of exertion, has some notoriety for its sheer physicality as a game. However, the sense of shared accomplishment that can be gained from playing the game well makes it worthwhile. Physical and strength differences between players can be managed by creating circles of children based on size, build and age.

Bull in the Ring

Playing this game well can be a breathless and exhilarating experience.

Organisation of players

The group make a circle with one volunteer – the bull – standing in the middle. Neighbours grip each other, interlocking hand and forearm, which should point up.

Playing the game

1   The bull must try to get out of the circle by breaking the grip of the players.

2   He must not use his hands, although he can push, shove and charge. He can also try to take the other players by surprise, appearing to charge one part of the circle but actually going for another.

3   The players in the circle must resist the bull, but they are not allowed to kick him.

4   When the bull manages to break the circle, another volunteer can take his place.

5   If a bull does not manage to break the circle, he can give up and another volunteer take his place.

Suggestion

An alternative way to play the game is for the bull to be on the outside of the ring. He must then break his way in. In yet another version, the ring contains a lamb (one child as volunteer) and it is a wolf on the outside that must break in. The circle then becomes the protector of the lamb.

Self-regulation

5 Games that focus attention

Self-regulation is about being able to focus one's attention and concentrate on something. This is achieved through a process of blocking out irrelevant stimuli in the environment and inhibiting unhelpful physical and mental impulses. Various methods are used here to help children develop this ability. These include physically making themselves wait for a signal, focusing on only one thing at a time and using visual cues to help organise attention in an activity. The final two games use a sophisticated 'delayed start', where children must inhibit the impulse to run until the start of the game has been called by another player.

Key terms

waiting, focusing on one thing, visual cue

Progression of skills

• wait for a cue – simple

• focus on one thing at a time

• use visual cues in a game

• wait for a cue – more advanced.

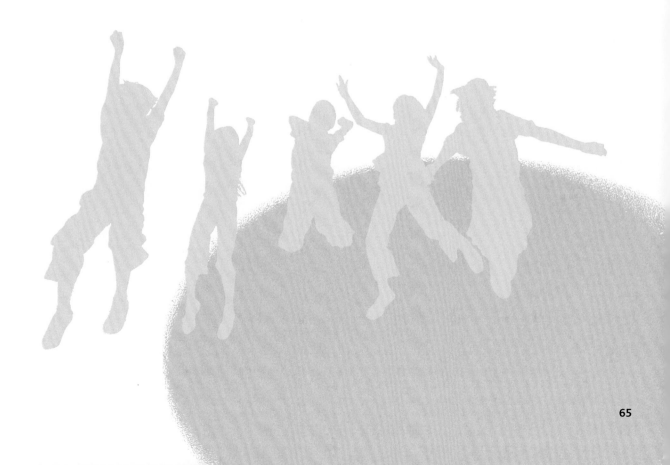

Clumps

This is an exciting game that requires children to wait for a signal by literally holding themselves together.

Organisation of players

Players spread themselves higgledy-piggledy around a large space. They curl up, face down, hugging their knees. One player, or an adult, acts as facilitator.

Playing the game

1   Instruct the group that when they are touched on the back, they are 'free'. This means the player can jump up and run round the room, weaving in and out of the other players as clumps.

2   Agree a signal to indicate that a player must stop running and go back to being a clump. For example, the signal could take the form of the facilitator holding up a red card.

3   With the players as clumps, the facilitator walks around the room eventually touching one child lightly on the back.

4   This player then runs around the room. It is possible for players to jump as well as run, jumping over the children as clumps.

5   At the signal, the player goes back to being a clump.

6   The facilitator continues walking around the room and touches another child.

Suggestion

For children who find it hard to remain as a clump, another child or an adult can support them by curling up beside them and putting an arm gently over their back. Some children find it hard to go back to being a clump when they are running around. In this case, the whole group can be called on to sit up, stay in their place but help 'shoo' the child back into a curled position.

Concentration

This game uses sight only and is especially good to play in the playground or another open space, although it can be played anywhere.

Organisation of players

Players sit round in or can stand in a circle.

Playing the game

1   Tell the players that they are going to play a game using only one of their senses, sight.

2   Instruct players to look around them for a set time, for example, a minute, and try to remember as many things as they can see. Players can be instructed to look for specific details such as objects or details of a particular shape or colour, or with a particular decoration.

3   When they are told to begin, players look for the set time and are then told to shut their eyes.

4   Each player must recall everything he has seen.

Suggestion

Playing the game one at a time, each player recalling immediately what he has seen, makes it simpler. An alternative focus for the game is hearing. Players are instructed to shut their eyes and listen for a set time, then open their eyes and list everything they have heard.

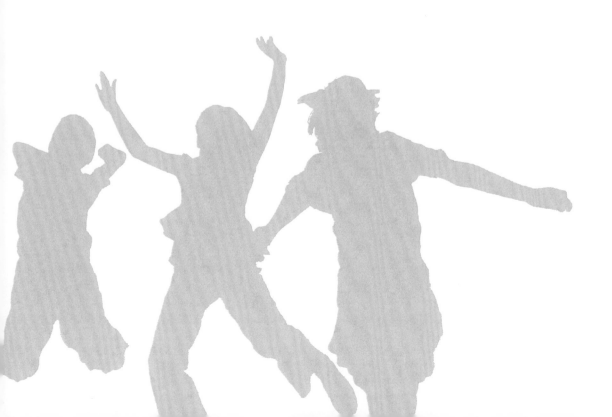

Feeling the Environment

This game focuses on touch as a sense.

Organisation of players

Players are put into pairs. One player is the leader, the other is blindfolded.

Playing the game

1 The leader takes her partner to an object or detail in the environment and puts his hands on it.

2 He feels the object, describes what he is feeling and guesses what the object or detail is.

3 The leader then takes him to another object to feel. Players can be required to find certain things, such as round objects, knobbly things, and so on.

4 Players swap roles, taking turns to be blindfolded.

Suggestion

Another way of playing the game is for familiar objects to be brought to players to feel or put in a feelie bag. A further alternative is to use taste instead of touch and ask blindfolded players to taste familiar foods and name them.

Sound Guide

This game encourages children to tune in to individual voices.

Organisation of players

The group is divided into pairs, with one partner blindfolded and the other being their sound guide.

Playing the game

1   In pairs, partners agree on their 'sound'. This is a noise, such as an animal sound, a funny sound or just a word, that the sound guide will use to lead his partner across the room.

2   Partners stand across the play space from each other. Players put on their blindfolds.

3   Sound guides start to make their agreed sound, remaining in one place.

4   Blindfolded players try to tune in to their sound and begin to walk towards their partner.

5   Sound guides are responsible for their partners and should use their sound to protect them as well as control them. For example, they should stop making their sound if the partner is about to bump into something or someone.

6   When partners find their sound guide, they give them feedback on how safe they made them feel.

Suggestion

The same effect of tuning in can be achieved through a whole-group activity. Children are organised into several groups of six or more. They make a tunnel by joining raised hands in pairs. For each tunnel, there is a blindfolded player. Tunnels begin to call out the name of their player. Blindfolded players move in the direction of their name, eventually going through their tunnel.

Think About!

Using visual cues

The term 'visual cue' means something that is visual – pictures, gestures and signs – used for the purposes of communication rather than decoration or stimulation of the imagination. We use visual cues all the time in our communication but are often unaware of the fact. When we are trying to communicate in another language, the use of visual cues is pronounced, with people using faces, hands, gestures, pointing and pictures to support what is not being communicated well verbally. In autism education, visual cues are commonly used for just this purpose, to make communication clearer when ordinary verbal communication is not that well understood.

Children, for whom verbal language is perhaps less important than it is for adults, frequently use visual cues in their play. Visual markers are sometimes used to demarcate areas of play, such as the lines of a football pitch or the bases of a rounders match. Natural markers are often used by children in play to denote boundaries or something strategic within a game, such as 'home'. The following are examples of the ways in which visual cues may be introduced into the playing of games:

- coloured flags or markers to indicate start (green) and stop (red)
- coloured cards held up to indicate wait (yellow) and stop (red)
- marks on the ground to indicate where to stand or run to
- who is 'It' being indicated by the player standing up, standing in a certain place, holding the ball, and so on
- the direction of play being indicated by the movement of the ball or the movement of players

Children think about:

Playing a game usually means that I have to stand in one place and move to another place. I can find out where I stand and where I move to by looking around me. I can also look to see where other players stand. I can look out for landmarks in the game, like a wall or a bench, to tell me where to go. Before a game starts I can ask the other children where I stand in a game and where I have to move to.

Ball Names

In this game, visual cues are used to indicate where players stand.

Organisation of players

Coloured markers are placed in a circle on the ground. Players stand on these. A different coloured marker is placed in the middle of the circle.

Playing the game

1   One player stands in the centre and bounces a ball on the ground. As she does so she calls out the name of another player.

2   She runs back to her place while the player she has called runs into the centre of the circle.

3   He must try to reach the ball before it bounces a given number of times or bounces out of the circle.

4   He stands in the centre and begins the game again by calling another player's name.

Suggestion

This game addresses the fact that children with autism are often not sure where to stand in a game or where to move to. Flat circles on the ground, chalked marks or any other kind of marking can be used in a game to indicate where a player stands and moves to.

Follow the Light

A visual cue is incorporated into this game to indicate where players should move to.

Organisation of players

One player has a torch with which he controls the group. The game must be played in the dark.

Playing the game

1   The player with the torch moves the beam around the play space.

2   The rest of the players try to 'catch' the beam of light by moving with it.

3   When the light rests on something, players try to 'tag' it by touching the light, using their hands or their feet.

4   When the light is tagged, that player takes the torch and the game begins again.

Suggestion

A long ribbon streamer can be used in the same way.

Obstacle Course

The obstacles in this game provide a clear indication of where players should move to next.

Organisation of players

Players agree on an obstacle course. Obstacles can require children to pull themselves along, roll across, jump over or crawl through and weave in and out. Where objects in the environment are being used, such as low walls or benches, mark these out as part of the course with flags.

Playing the game

1 Players are shown what they have to do in the obstacle course.

2 They line up to take their turn and go when they are instructed to.

3 Some players may stand along the course to assist the others through the obstacle or remind them what to do.

Suggestion

There is great flexibility about making obstacle courses. They can be created indoors or out, and use special equipment or objects that just happen to be there. They can also be enjoyed in different settings: in school, in the park or at home. For even greater clarity in the game, obstacles can be numbered '1, 2, 3...' to indicate where to go next.

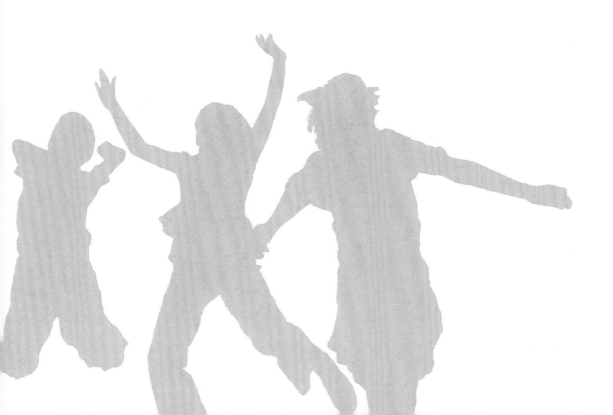

Doorways

The position of the players' arms, making doorways through which children pass, provides the visual cue in this game.

Organisation of players

Players stand or sit in a circle. By joining hands and raising their arms, they make 'doorways' in the spaces in-between.

Playing the game

1   One child is chosen and stands in the middle of the circle.

2   She weaves her way in and out of the circle by going in and out of the doorways, moving round the circle of players as she does so.

3   When she has gone round the whole circle, she joins the circle again.

4   Another player is chosen to go through the doorways.

Suggestion

The game can be varied by having more than one player go through the doorways. Children can go in the same direction or different directions. As a way of adding further challenge, doorways can be made smaller or narrower.

In and Out the Dusty Bluebells

This is very similar to the previous game, but with the addition of a ritual and a song. Players must wait to be selected to join in the dance.

Organisation of players

Players stand in a circle and hold hands. Hands are raised in the air to form arches.

Playing the game

1 One player volunteers to go first and stands in the centre of the circle.

2 This player weaves her way in and out of the circle, going through the arches the other players have made. As she does so, the children sing:

   In and out the dusty bluebells

   In and out the dusty bluebells

   In and out the dusty bluebells

   Who will be my partner?

3 At the end of this chorus, the player taps the nearest child and says 'You will be my partner'.

4 This player becomes the new leader and the first child stands behind him with her hands on his shoulders or waist. The new leader continues to weave in and out of the circle as the chorus is sung again.

5 New leaders continue to be chosen in this way, with the line of players going in and out of the circle getting longer, until only two players remain to make a single arch.

Suggestion

As the snaking line of players gets longer, the game becomes increasingly exciting for players, making it hard for them to control their impulses. Holding hands in the circle encourages players to wait their turn.

Ready, Steady, Go!

This is less of a game and more an activity to practise children's skills in coping with a delayed start.

Organisation of players

Arrange different activities for the group to carry out, such as building something, racing over a distance or going round an obstacle course. Choose activities that all players are reasonably good at.

Playing the game

1   Tell players that they are going to have fun with 'Ready, steady, go!'.

2   Use the different activities you have set out to practise starting the activity. Try different methods of conveying the start, for example, ringing a bell, blowing a whistle or simply saying 'Ready, steady, go'.

3   Discuss with players how it feels to wait for the start of a game and how hard they find it.

4   Practise it a few times to see if players improve.

5   Let players take turns to be the person who starts an activity.

Suggestion

Some games have a delayed start, where players wait to be told to begin playing. A delayed start to a game can mean a great build-up of tension and challenges all players to wait for 'Go!'.

Self-regulation

6 Exciting games

Children with autism love to be chased, but the chasing can become endless with the child running over a large area, never allowing themselves to be caught. This kind of endless chasing exemplifies the fact that children with autism often get lost in the intoxicating feeling of playing exciting games with little overall sense of a social structure inherent in what they are doing and where they are going.

These next games all involve some kind of chasing and catching, but include ideas about how to introduce structure to help children know what is expected of them and cope better with the feeling of excitement. It can be helpful to point out something about excitement as an emotion: that it is a strong feeling which is sometimes difficult to control. The first game simply focuses on the fact that a game has both a start and a finish. After this, different ways of providing structure in games are given. These include having clear play boundaries for a game, introducing simple rules and introducing pretend sequences that children must follow. The final two games test children's capacity to cope with the excitement that comes with a delayed start.

Key terms

starting, finishing, keeping to a rule, the feeling of excitement

Progression of skills

• understand that games start and finish

• keep to boundaries within a game

• keep to a rule

• cope with suspense in a game.

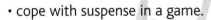

I'm Coming to Get You!

Use this game to emphasise the fact that a game has both a beginning and an ending.

Organisation of players

Players form pairs consisting of a child and an adult, or a younger child and an older child.

Playing the game

1 The adult or older child announces in a playful way 'I'm coming to get you!' and indicates that the other player should run away.

2 She chases after him, calling out every so often 'I'm coming to get you!'.

3 When the younger child is caught, the catcher announces playfully 'I've got you!'.

4 The game is played again.

Suggestion

This game should be played in as enjoyable a way as possible, with the focus on two people having fun together. If it is very difficult to catch the child, 'I've got you!' can be said later, at the first convenient moment. Do not worry too much about reversing roles, with the child doing the chasing.

Duck, Duck, Goose

Here the organisation of the players in a circle clearly defines where to run.

Organisation of players

Players sit in a circle.

Playing the game

1 One player is chosen to walk round the outside of the circle.

2 He touches each player on the shoulder, naming each one 'Duck'.

3 After a while he names one player 'Goose!' and begins to run round the circle.

4 The player who has been named jumps up and chases after him.

5 The first player tries to go all the way round the circle and sit in the empty space without being caught. If he does so, the new player begins the game again.

6 If the player who is 'Goose' manages to catch him, the first player must start again going round the circle.

Suggestion

A clear indication of where to carry out an activity may be an important piece of information for a child. An activity may confuse a child with autism simply in terms of where they are expected to do it – from where, to where, and so on – rather than the actual action or interaction involved.

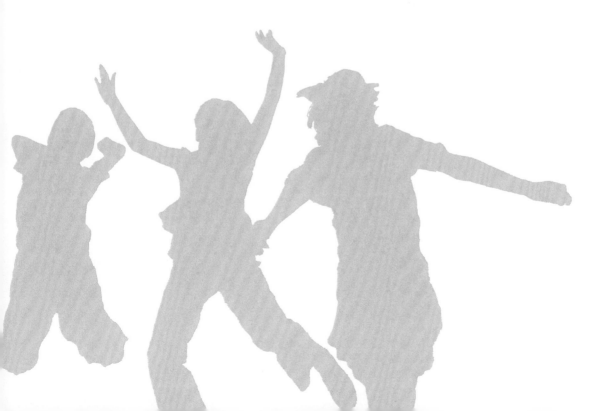

Crossing Over

The natural boundaries of the play space are used to define where to run from and to. This game can be used in conjunction with any form of tag game.

Organisation of players

Players line up against a wall facing another wall some distance away. One player is 'It' and stands facing the others mid-way between the two walls.

Playing the game

1   When he is ready, the player in the middle shouts out 'Cross over!'

2   Players against the wall run across the play space to the wall on the other side, which is safety.

3   The player in the middle tries to tag players as they cross.

4   When a player is tagged, she must sit out of the game.

Suggestion

Instead of crossing between walls, it is possible to use any natural boundary to the play space, such as buildings, pavements or trees. Clearly marked boundaries work best, however. Using painted playground lines, for example, gives rise to disputes about which line is being used in the game.

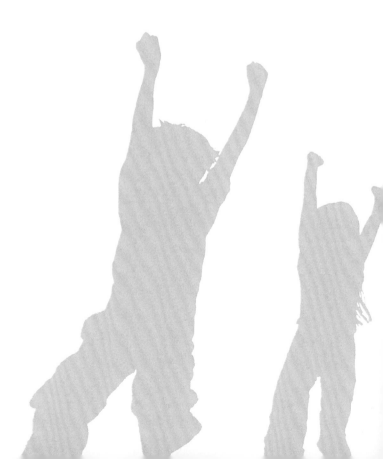

Fox and Geese

This game is played on an outline marked on the ground.

Organisation of players

Mark a circle on the ground in chalk measuring approximately three metres in diameter.
Draw out eight equal sections, with lines coming out from the centre of the circle like the spokes of a wheel. One player is the fox and stands in the centre of the circle. All the other players are geese and position themselves along the rim of the circle.

Playing the game

1   The fox starts to chase the geese. All the players, fox and geese, can run in any direction but must stay on the lines at all times.

2   When two geese meet each other they may pass but must manoeuvre round each other carefully, keeping their feet on the lines of the circle.

3   When the fox catches a goose, she tags him, which means that he must sit out of the game.

4   Play continues until one goose is left.

Suggestion

Consider how other familiar games can be marked out visually in this way.

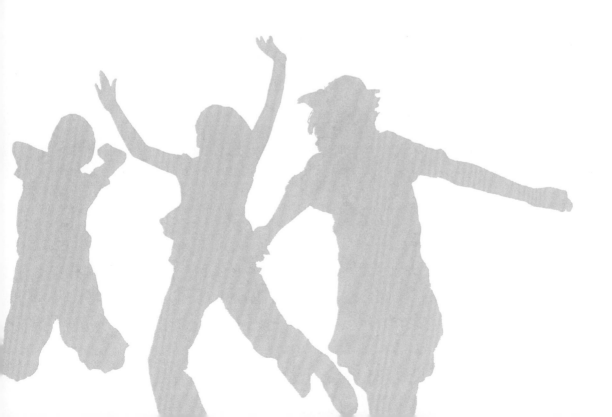

Think About!

Being 'It'

The large amount of running, chasing and dodging in games of tag can prohibit many children with autism from playing and enjoying them. Being 'It' is difficult for many children, with or without autism, since it requires a child to be a good runner, sufficiently fit to run over a distance. Yet tag games are perennially popular in schools among children of different ages. What is being offered here, therefore, is different ways of thinking about being 'It' and a number of alternatives to playing the traditional game of Tag.

Children's games use different forms of 'It'. 'It' can have little power in a game and weak control over the other players. The 'It' in games such as Tag is weak since the child must chase others endlessly, having little power to stop them or control their movement. A much more powerful 'It' is found in the game 'What's the Time, Mr Wolf?' where 'It', just by turning round, causes players to start and stop. By adjusting a game slightly, it is possible to move a weak 'It' towards being more powerful and thereby giving the player more control and satisfaction in playing the game. Alternative ways of playing Tag that are more accessible to children who are not good runners and dodgers thus involve adjusting the balance of power between players by making 'It' more powerful.

Children think about:

I can choose how I want to be 'It':

- children, except for me, have to hop, jump or move in another way that is not fast running

- I can tag using long scarves or by throwing a soft ball

- children have to touch something as they run to safety – I can stand near whatever it is and tag them as they touch it or step on it

- children must not touch the ground – they have to walk on walls or benches, or stay in a tree.

Frisbee Game

This is a tag game that gives more power to the player who is 'It'.

Organisation of players

As for 'Crossing Over' (see page 80), players line up against one end of the play space. One player who is 'It' stands mid-way holding a frisbee.

Playing the game

1 On the instruction of the player who is 'It', players begin to run to the other side of the play space.

2 The player catches them by throwing the frisbee. If the frisbee hits any part of a player, she must sit out of the game.

3 Players must cross the play space an agreed number of times or until all the players have been caught out.

Suggestion

Hard plastic frisbees can hurt when they hit a player, but soft frisbees that are just as effective and easier to throw are available on the market.

Three Lives

The rule here is that a player can have more than one chance before they are out of the game.

Organisation of players

The game begins with players standing in a circle.

Playing the game

1   One player throws a soft ball into the circle. Whoever it touches or comes to rest beside picks it up while all the other players begin to run.

2   The player with the ball throws it at another player.

3   If it touches him, he loses a life.

4   The player who is then nearest the ball picks it up and throws it at another player, trying to hit them. When players have the ball, they must not move with it.

5   The play continues, with players nearest the ball throwing it, until all players have lost their three lives.

Suggestion

This game has the advantage that no player need be 'It' for very long.

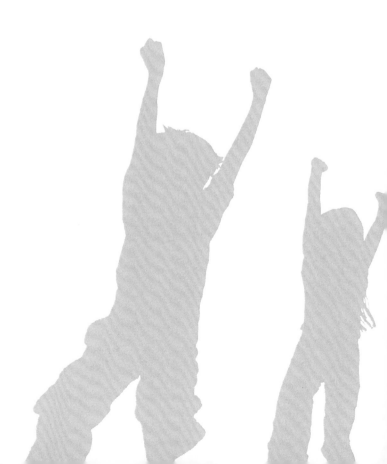

Touchwood

Touchwood introduces the idea that a player can make himself safe from being caught by touching something.

Organisation of players

The game begins by players running at will from the child who is 'It'.

Playing the game

1   Players run to any object that is made of wood and touch it. When they do so they are safe from being caught by the player who is 'It'.

2   Players can taunt the child who is 'It' when they are standing near safety, calling attention to themselves by saying:

> *Tiggy, tiggy, touch wood,*
>
> *I'm not touching wood!*

3   Players are not allowed to stay in any one place for very long and must run to find other wood to touch.

4   When players are caught they are out, and when all players are caught the game is over, unless 'It' has already given up.

Suggestion

Other forms of sanctuary can be found, such as touching metal, touching a colour, being off the ground or getting into groups of two, three or four.

Touchwood is a good example of a game where 'It' is very low powered. It can be pointed out to children that some chasing games are more about having fun with teasing the chaser than about catching other players.

Stepping Stones

Introducing an element of pretence can increase the excitement levels in a game.

Organisation of players

Play the game near walls, benches or some other kind of raised area. One player is 'It'. She adopts the role of something that is threatening, such as a monster, zombie or shark. She moves around on the ground freely. All the other players must try to stay above ground.

Playing the game

1   The player who is 'It' moves around the space pretending to be threatening.

2   Players also move around the play space, but if they touch the ground they can be caught by being tagged.

3   When a player is caught, he is ritualistically removed to a 'prison' area where he must remain.

Suggestion

Children's games often include a contemporary theme, such as the latest popular television programme, film or toy. These can be used to inspire the choice of roles in this game, using any two oppositional characters or groups.

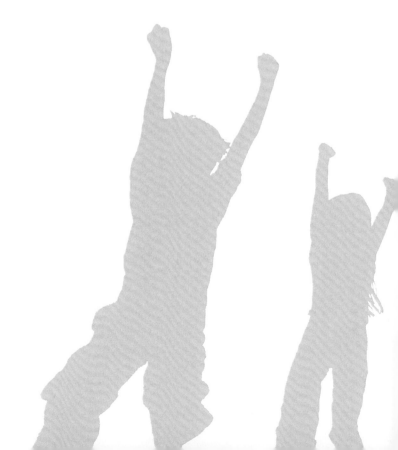

Crusts and Crumbs

Suspense is heightened here by delaying the start of this game and hanging on to the 'crrr' of 'crusts' or 'crumbs'.

Organisation of players

The group is divided into two sides, 'Crusts' and 'Crumbs', facing each other two metres across a space of roughly two metres. They are equidistant from two boundaries marking the point to which players must run for safety. One player is a caller.

Playing the game

1 The caller calls out either 'Crusts' or 'Crumbs'.

2 Whichever side is called must chase the other side, who run to the boundary behind them.

3 Players who are caught before they reach safety must join the other side.

4 The two sides line up and the game is played again.

Suggestion

Playing games with delayed starts practises the ability to control impulses and inhibit actions. Choose a good caller and have fun with delaying the start of games, repeating the activity so that children improve at waiting for a signal.

Poison

Suspense is heightened by the delayed start as well as players close proximity to the child who is 'It'.

Organisation of players

The player who is 'It' holds out her hands with fingers spread. Players take hold of a finger, stretching as far away from her as they can and preparing to run.

Playing the game

1   The player who is 'It' says 'I went to the shops and I bought some …', naming a food item. The player continues, repeating the same sentence and naming other items. She can tease players by naming items that begin with 'p' and playing with this, for example, 'I went to the shops and I bought a bottle of p-p-p-Pepsi'.

2   When the player who is 'It' says 'I went to the shops and I bought a bottle of poison!', this is the signal for players to run.

3   The player who is 'It' chases them and tries to tag them.

4   If a player runs before the signal, he must become 'It' and begin the game again.

5   When a player is tagged, he must freeze in one place until another player releases him by crawling through his legs.

Suggestion

Any sentence and signal word can be used in this game. Let children invent their own versions and play that game together.

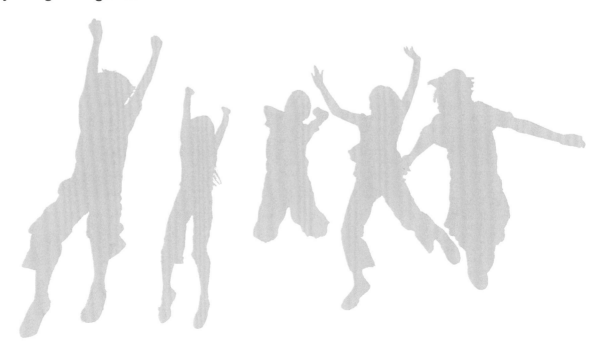

Adapting to others

When children adapt themselves to the play of others in games, they coordinate their actions and responses as well as share play ideas. They give up some of what is theirs – their responses, their ideas and their interests – for the sake of maintaining a situation of play with other children. Adapting to others suggests more than simple cooperation. It is not simply interacting, but taking on the ideas and interests of someone else and creating something new together. Children with autism often find this kind of adaptation difficult. They tend to be more fixed in terms of their interests, less willing to give up their own ideas and unable to see other points of view.

Research shows that peers are instrumental in the social integration of children with autism, but in thinking about how to support children with autism and their peers, it is important to be clear about what involvement really consists of in children's social worlds. For all children, interaction, play and friendship are less about fixed internal ideas and more about an interpersonal working out of those things that happens over time between groups of children. In particular, children's social worlds are marked out by their emotionality. Enjoying each other's company and having fun together leads to greater knowledge and understanding of other people. It is the emotional quality of the engagement that promotes trust and the willingness to give up one's own interests and sort out differences for the sake of the game. Adapting to others is about enjoying being with others, taking pleasure in what you do together and wanting it to continue. The games here maximise the experience of enjoyment that can be had when playing together, with the emphasis on games that are fun to play, and promote laughter and mutual satisfaction.

Adapting to others

7 Mutual enjoyment through games

All children, including children with autism, interact more effectively the more they enjoy the experience. For a child who is unsure and wary of other people, an important piece of learning is that it is possible to take pleasure in the company of others. For effective social skills learning this must come first, before any idea of adapting to other children, taking on their ideas and points of view, and collaborating on something together.

These next games are about promoting the experience of enjoyment that can be had in group activity. They are organised into games that involve pairs or small groups of players and games that promote whole-group fun. Some children may find whole-group experiences overwhelming, so being able to play in a pair or a group of three may be a better place to start. The final games in this section are about children collaborating together in an enjoyable way to create funny whole-group mimes.

Key terms

having fun together, smiling at each other, laughing together

Progression of skills

• have fun in a pair or small group

• have fun as a whole group

• whole-group mimes.

Think About!

Winning and losing

There is a difference between children's games and games that are devised by adults. Adult-created games tend to be competitive, with the outcome usually being a situation of winners and losers. For children, the most important thing is playing, and although their games may have a competitive element, they are much more concerned with keeping the play going. Winners and losers are less important, and competition even becomes problematic if it dominates the game so that players drop out. Children tend to be inclusive in their games, adaptable to the needs of as many players as possible. Children's games are good at taking account of the differences between players, and traditionally are played by children of different ages.

For children with autism, the issue of winning and losing in play can be highly problematic. Some children feel they must win in a game because to lose means they are 'wrong' in some way. But winning itself often gives a child little satisfaction. Children may be offered explanations about 'fairness' or 'equality' in play, but this is not strictly logical in terms of competitive games. Alternatively, there is the 'probability approach', where children are told that they can only reasonably expect to win a certain number of times given the number of players involved. Whichever way the issue is tackled, however, the issue of winning and losing remains a difficult one for many children.

Sometimes it is better to focus on non-competitive games. Adapting to others works two ways. Where a child is experiencing difficulty with competitive play, the group may need to adapt to that child. In fact, the preferences of children in a group are never all the same but it is certain that what suits one will also appeal to others.

Children think about:

If playing competitive games means that we have lots of arguments, we can decide to play more games that are non-competitive. Non-competitive games are fun to play, but do not have one person being the winner and everyone else losing. We can try out playing non-competitively to see if we would like to play more non-competitive games.

Group Numbers

This is a whole-group activity that involves players making a connection with only a small group of players at a time.

Organisation of players

Players walk around a large play space. One player is the caller and stands to one side.

Playing the game

1 Players walk freely around the play area.

2 The caller gives them the instruction to form groups of a given number of players. He does this by calling out 'Make twos!' He can instruct players to make any size group: 'Make threes!', 'Make fours!', and so on.

3 When the caller instructs them, players must make a group of that size as quickly as they can, finding the right number of players and standing together.

4 The caller checks that the groups have been established properly. If this is the case, he shouts 'Walk on!' and the game begins again.

Suggestion

This game is often played more competitively, with players having to sit out of the game if they cannot find a group, and one player eventually becoming the winner. However, the game is perhaps more enjoyable for children if played non-competitively.

Mousetrap

This is a game for five players.

Organisation of players

A large square is drawn out on the ground, with two diagonal lines and a small circle in the middle. One player is 'It' and stands in the circle. The other players stand in the four corners of the square

Playing the game

1   The player who is 'It' must try to get to one of the corners. The other four players must work together to prevent this from happening.

2   Players can make eye contact, nod and gesture to each other, but they must not speak. Any two players can swap corners, running along the lines of the square or across the diagonal. However, they must do so without 'It' getting into their corner.

3   When players swap corners, the player who is 'It' tries to move into that corner.

4   When a player is left without a corner, she becomes 'It' and stands in the centre of the square.

Suggestion

The visual element of lines along which to run sets out a clear expectation of what to do in the game.

Sardines

This is a hunting game played more for fun than for the purpose of winning.

Organisation of players

A few of the players go to hide themselves while the rest of the group close their eyes.

Playing the game

1   The players with their eyes closed count to 30.

2   One player opens her eyes and goes off to look for a hidden player.

3   While she is looking, the remaining players close their eyes and count to 30 again.

4   When the player who is seeking finds a hider, she joins him in the hiding place instead of giving him away.

5   If she cannot find a hidden player, she simply hides herself.

6   When the players have finished counting, another player goes off to look for hiders while another 30 is counted.

7   Play continues in this way until there are no more players to count.

Suggestion

This game can be played competitively with players being 'out' if they cannot find a player. However, the real fun of the game is in the sharing of a hiding place, and the laughter that usually ensues. For this reason, good hiding places, such as behind a large curtain or under a slide, are important. If necessary, hiding places can be pointed out to children before the game starts.

1–15

This is a very simple game to play as a whole group.

Organisation of players

Players sit higgledy-piggledy on chairs or on the ground.

Playing the game

1 The group must count from 1 to 15 with players taking it in turns to say a number. However, players do not know whose turn it is – turns are not indicated by going round the circle, for example.

2 The counting proceeds by players calling out a number.

3 If two players call out at the same time, the whole group must start counting again.

Suggestion

There are lots of versions of this game. The number to which players count can be determined by the number of members in the group. Counting can be forwards or backwards. Players can play the game as a countdown, counting down from 10 to 1 and shouting 'Lift off!' together at the end.

Group Juggling

With practice, this game can provide a satisfying whole-group experience.

Organisation of players

Players stand higgledy-piggledy around the play space. Two or more balls are needed for the game.

Playing the game

1 One player begins the game by throwing a ball to another player.

2 That player must throw the ball to a third player, who throws it to a fourth.

3 The ball continues around the group, each player choosing a new player to whom to throw the ball.

4 Eventually, the ball will return to the player who first threw it. This establishes the route the ball must take through the group and remains fixed for the whole game.

5 The ball is thrown again around the group, following the same route. This is done a few times.

6 Once the first ball is being juggled by the group with ease, a second, third and even fourth ball can be gradually introduced. Each time, the first player throws in the new ball and it is juggled by the group following the same sequence of players.

Suggestion

Soft balls and koosh balls are easier to catch and can be used in this game.

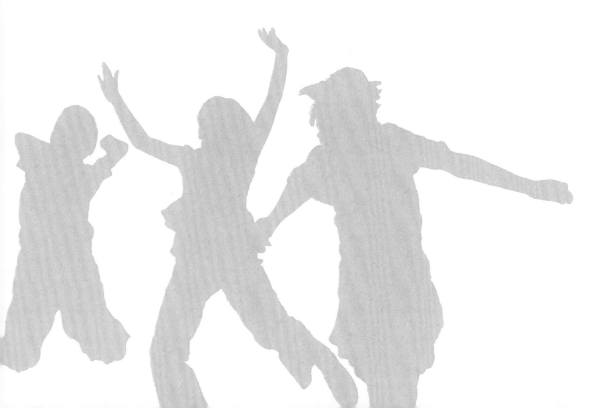

Floaters

This is a perfect game for whole-group fun.

Organisation of players

Players sit in chairs higgledy-piggledy around the play space. There is one empty chair.

Playing the game

1   One person volunteers to be 'It' and stands at the edge of the play space, on the opposite side to the empty chair.

2   The player must try to sit down in the empty chair and begins to walk at a steady pace towards it.

3   The other players must work together to prevent the player who is 'It' from sitting in the empty chair.

4   They can move from chair to chair, sitting in an empty chair as 'It' approaches.

5   When the player who is 'It' manages to sit down, another player becomes 'It' and the game begins again.

Suggestion

It is tempting for the player who is 'It' to speed up as they move towards an empty chair, rushing to sit down. Players should be instructed that they have to maintain a steady pace when they are 'It'.

Gobbling Goblins!

This is an acting game that involves trying not to laugh.

Organisation of players

Three players volunteer to be the goblins and stand away from the play space. An area is designated as the goblins' house.

Playing the game

1　All players except the goblins go into the house and look round.

2　It is agreed beforehand that one player will shout out a warning signal, such as 'Watch out, the goblins are coming back!'

3　At this signal, everyone must freeze. The goblins will not eat them if they can stay still, pretending to be a piece of furniture or a wall.

4　The goblins return to their house and start to sniff around.

5　They test the players by trying to make them laugh. They can do anything that is funny but they must not touch a player.

6　If a player laughs, he gives away the fact that he is not an object and so can be eaten by the goblin.

Suggestion

In designating the goblins' house, it is possible to base the imaginative play on concrete objects in the play space with, for example, a bench as the goblins' sofa, a bunker for their oven, and so on.

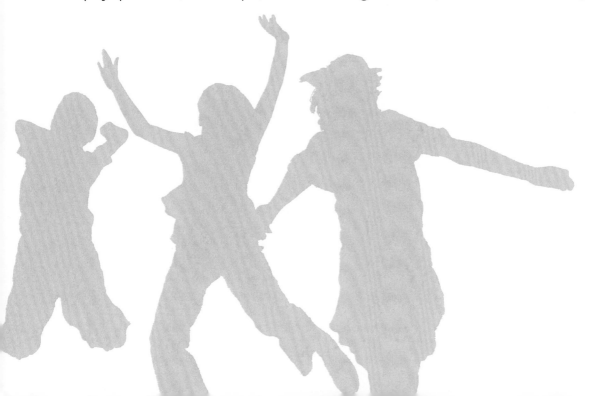

Let's Do It

In this game, players create mimed actions in a group.

Organisation of players

Players walk around freely within the play space. They listen out for instructions about what actions to perform.

Playing the game

1   Any player can name an action to perform. For example, the action might be 'Jump three times', 'Touch our toes' or 'Walk like a penguin'.

2   At the beginning of the game, any player can start by calling out an instruction, saying 'Let's ...' and giving the action.

3   When an instruction is called, all players stop where they are and call back 'Yes, let's!' Everyone in the group then mimes that action.

4   Players continue to walk around the space listening out for the next instruction.

5   Another player calls out an instruction.

Suggestion

Instructions can be as elaborate and imaginative as players want them to be and can easily incorporate the special interests of a child with autism. Players might suggest 'Let's jump like Spiderman' or 'Let's get zapped by radiation!'

There Ain't No Flies ...

In this game, players chant a refrain to an opposing side.

Organisation of players

The group divides and stands in two lines, quite far apart, facing each other.

Playing the game

1   One line of players steps forward and says:

> *There ain't no flies on us*
>
> *There ain't no flies on us*
>
> *There may be flies on you guys*
>
> *But there ain't no flies on us.*

2   The players in this line stay where they are as the second line steps forward and repeats the refrain back to them.

3   Taking it in turns, the two lines of players proceed in this way, taking a step forward and repeating the refrain.

4   Each time the refrain is spoken, the players get louder and more menacing.

5   When the two lines meet in the middle, players can put their arms in the air and hug or shake hands with the players on the other side, at whom they have just been shouting.

Suggestion

There is antagonism in this game, but no competition as such. Children can put more feeling into saying the lines by putting their hands on their hips and pointing in an accusing way at the other players.

Lemonade

This game involves a group refrain accompanied by a mime.

Organisation of players

The group divide into two teams and stand in two lines facing each other.

Playing the game

1   One team, Team A, decides among themselves what 'trade' they are. They can be 'carpenters from Clapham', 'truck drivers from Trowbridge', 'nurses from Neath', and so on.

2   When they have decided on a trade and how to mime it, they line up ready, facing the other side.

3   The two sides chant the following lines to each other:

> Team B: *Where are you from?*
>
> Team A: *Clapham*
>
> Team B: *What's your trade?*
>
> Team A: *Lemonade*
>
> Team B: *Show us your trade if you're not afraid*
>
> Team A: *We're not afraid to show you our trade.*

4   Team A members then carry out their mimes, for example, miming carpentry.

5   Team B watch and try to guess what the trade is, knowing that it must begin with the same initial letter as the location given.

6   When they guess correctly, the game begins again with the two sides swapping roles.

Suggestion

This repartee is a prelude to a chase, where the second team chases the first back to their starting point behind them as soon as they have guessed correctly, but it is sufficiently enjoyable to play without this.

Adapting to others

8 Games that avoid conflict

Sometimes, children's play has nothing to do with conflict or competition and is much more about showing you care about someone else, looking after others and tending to their needs. Typically, such play is characteristic of girls' play, but boys too can be witnessed taking part in such activity. The first three games outlined here involve players looking after each other and making something pleasurable for someone else to enjoy. For children with autism, these games should definitely make use of their special interests. The following four games require players to copy the actions and expressions of other children and so show an interest in them and what they do. The final games are about players being protective of other players, taking care that another player is not hurt and keeping them safe in the game.

Key terms

looking after others, copying, taking care

Progression of skills

• care for another child

• copy another child

• protect others when playing.

Rocking

This game requires some equipment, for example, a hammock or a swing chair.

Organisation of players

A number of players elect to be rocked. As many as can fit comfortably should sit in the hammock or chair.

Playing the game

1   The remaining players stand around the hammock and begin to rock it gently.

2   They must take care not to bump it against their legs or any posts.

3   As they rock the players, they ask for feedback, such as whether they should rock more gently or a little faster.

4   The players in the hammock should be given enough time to relax and enjoy the sensation of rocking before they swap over and let other players have a turn.

Suggestion

Pieces of equipment such as a hammock or swing chair are much less expensive to buy than they used to be. They can be kept in a cupboard and brought out occasionally to give children a treat or can be a more permanent feature of a play space.

Building Dens

This game is about building a nice environment for another player to enjoy.

Organisation of players

One or two players sit out while the other players work together to build a den.

Playing the game

1   The player or players for whom the den is intended are questioned about their preferences. For example, they can be asked if they want a roof, somewhere to sit or lie down, windows, an interesting way of entering, and so on.

2   The players who are making the den discuss how they are going to build it and look around for objects they can use to make it.

3   Players build the den using found objects. They can also use themselves in the structure, to make walls, seats and doors.

4   Once the den is ready, the players for whom it is intended enter it and enjoy it for a while.

Suggestion

Dens can be as elaborate as players want them to be. They can have music and sound effects, pictures on the walls, machinery and technology, all made by the other players. For children with autism, make sure to incorporate any special interests they may have to maximise their enjoyment.

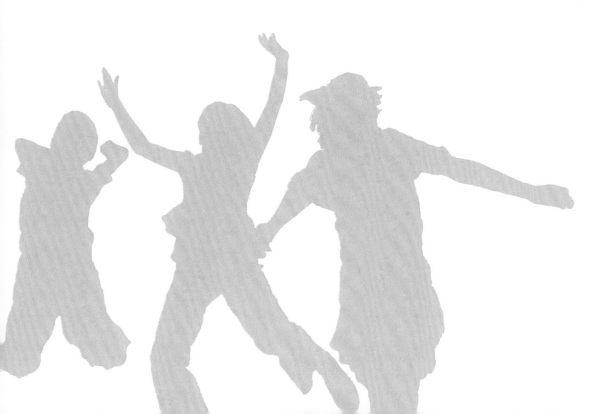

Through the Rushes

Children provide a pleasant sensory experience for a player.

Organisation of players

Players divide into two lines and make a tunnel, standing a metre apart and facing each other. One child at a time elects to go 'through the rushes'.

Playing the game

1 The child who is going to go through the rushes stands at one end of the two lines of players.

2 He is blindfolded or simply closes his eyes and begins to walk through the tunnel of players.

3 As he does so, the players give him a pleasant sensory experience, brushing against him gently with their fingers, blowing softly, making soothing noises – whatever they can think to do to give a pleasant sensation.

4 The child emerges from the tunnel and tells the others how it felt.

5 Another child elects to go through the rushes.

Suggestion

For some children, it is a pleasant experience to hear their name softly said as well as they go through the tunnel. Others may prefer to be led slowly down the tunnel rather than find their own way. Be sure to use children's special interests in making a pleasant experience.

Crossed Wires

This is an 'echo' game where one player's movements are copied by the whole group.

Organisation of players

The group stand in a circle.

Playing the game

1 One player looks at another player across the circle.

2 That player then focuses on a third player across from him.

3 The third player focuses on another and so on until all the players have someone with whom they are connected.

4 Once this has been established, the players should not move. However, if someone does move, the player who is looking at him should copy what he does.

5 This movement will then be copied around the circle.

Suggestion

If simply looking is not a clear enough indication of which player is linked to which, players can point at the player to whom they are connecting.

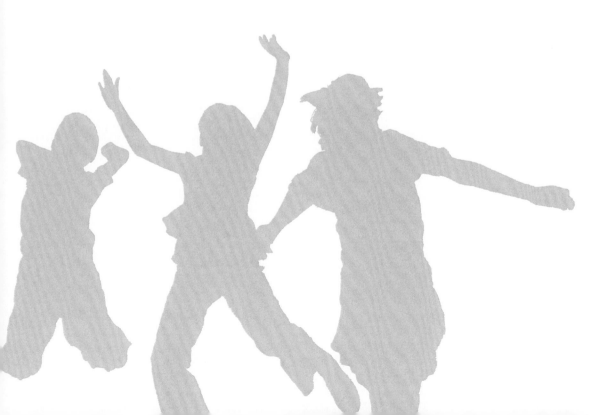

Addabout

This is a simple circle game where players copy each other's actions and add one of their own.

Organisation of players

Players stand or sit in a circle.

Playing the game

1 One player starts by making a simple movement, such as twiddling his thumbs, stamping his foot, or giving a 'high five' to the air.

2 The player next to him repeats the action and then adds another action of her own.

3 The player next to her does the same, adding a third action.

4 The game continues in this way round the circle, getting progressively more difficult as players have to recall more and more actions.

5 When the game has gone round the whole circle, the first player must perform all the actions starting with his original action.

Suggestion

Another way of playing this is as a name game with children saying their name, or even the sentence 'I'm Tom and here's my sound', inserting their name. This sentence and the sound then have to be copied. Players can choose a movement or sound that relates to something in which they are particularly interested.

Clapping Rhythms

This is a clapping game that reverberates across the whole group.

Organisation of players

Players stand or sit in a circle.

Playing the game

1 One player, Player A, is the leader and claps or makes some other sound.

2 The player to her right, Player B, copies the sound.

3 The player to the left of the leader, Player C, then copies the sound.

4 The sound then jumps back across the circle to the player on the right of Player B, then back again to the player on the left of Player C.

5 The sound reverberates across the circle this way until all the players have had a turn.

6 Before the sound reaches the last player, the leader may begin a new sound so that more than one rhythm is going across the circle at any one time.

Suggestion

For a less formal way of playing this game, players can sit haphazardly, first establishing a route for the clapping by players taking it in turns to clap. New rhythms can still be introduced by a lead player while a sound is being passed around the group.

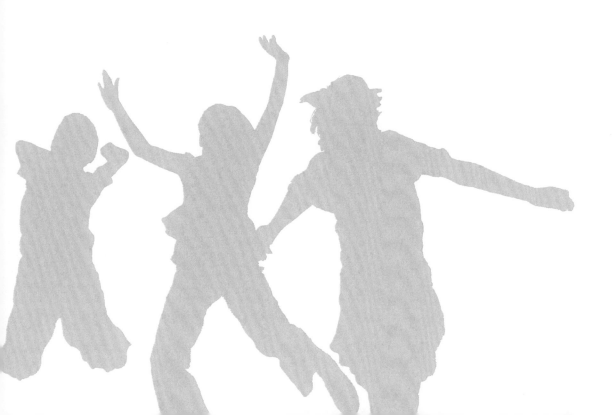

The Vortex

Players follow each other in a line to make a 'vortex' in the centre of the play space.

Organisation of players

Players hold hands in a circle. One player is the leader.

Playing the game

1 Holding hands with only one neighbour, the leader breaks the circle and begins to lead the line of players around the room.

2 She follows a wide arc initially but gradually leads the players into a spiral path, spiralling into the centre of the play space.

3 Once the vortex has been made, the leader doubles back by walking between the lines of players.

4 She leads the players back into the circle, ending as they had started.

5 Another player opts to be the leader.

Suggestion

Leading a large group of players needs to be slowly and thoughtfully done. Enough space must be allowed for children to move. Creating a tight spiral, however, does usually give rise to lots of laughter.

Think About!

Children's peer cultures

Children create their own cultures, influenced in part by the dominant adult culture and in part by their own interests, thoughts and personalities. Children create different kinds of cultures too. Gender, for example, will determine to some extent what children are like together. A group dominated by boys may favour interaction in large groups orientated towards physical games. If dominated by girls, however, a peer group may do more social activity in small groups and have stronger emotional attachments. Peer cultures can also be described in terms of their dynamic — whether there is mostly harmony or lots of bickering — and the degree to which the group look for 'sameness' in constituent members or tolerate difference. Peer cultures favour certain types of activities: physical games, competitive games, imaginative games, and so on.

When thinking about how to support the social engagement of children, an important consideration is the *culture* of the group. What are these children like as a group? What peer culture is dominant? This will determine to some extent whether to you should introduce a different cultural activity, say, non-competitive games to children who generally play sport.

Children think about:

What type of group are we? Answer the following:

• What sort of games do we play, eg running, pretending?

• Do we play the same game or different games?

• Do we play in a big group or in smaller groups?

• Do we fall out a lot?

• Is everyone the same in our group, or is it OK to be different, eg girls and boys?

All Fall Down

This is a cooperative game that requires each player to have a metre-long stick with which to play the game.

Organisation of players

Players stand higgledy-piggledy, standing no more than a stride away from another player. Each player has a stick which they stand on the ground in front of them, keeping it upright by touching it lightly on the top with their finger. One player is a caller.

Playing the game

1   The object of the game is for players to move without letting sticks fall to the ground.

2   At a signal, the players move to another stick, trying to reach it before it falls to the ground.

3   Each time the caller gives the signal, players must move to another stick trying to keep it upright.

Suggestion

If players find this variation of the game too easy, it can be made more difficult by introducing the rule that they have to miss out one staff and catch the next one, or by increasing the distance between players.

Circle of Knots

Players take care of each other as they create a tangled circle.

Organisation of players

Players join hands to form a ring.

Playing the game

1 One player begins by moving forward across the circle, under the hands of the players opposite. As he does this, the players who are holding his hands follow him, bringing other players with them.

2 A second player now makes a move, moving slowly and carefully and bringing the players she is holding on to with her.

3 Players continue to move in this way until as many 'knots' in the circle have been made and it seems as if no more movement is possible.

4 Players must move slowly, carefully and thoughtfully to ensure that no player is hurt in making the circle of knots. Players will need to adjust their grip, loosening or tightening it to allow movement, but without letting go.

5 Once the circle of knots is made, players begin to unravel it and get back into their original position without letting go of hands.

Suggestion

An alternative way of playing this game is for all players to start in the centre of the play space. They shut their eyes and put both hands out. They feel for two hands to hold. Then, with eyes open, players try to disentangle the knots they have made without letting hands go.

Streets and Alleys

In this game, players make a course by joining their hands and protect a player from being caught.

Organisation of players

This games requires at least 15 players to make the streets and alleys. There is also a chaser, a player who is chased and a caller. To create the course for the game, the players make three equal-sized groups and join hands with arms outstretched. They stand in three parallel rows about two metres apart to form 'streets'. The caller stands at the end of one of the streets.

Playing the game

1   The player who is chasing starts at one end of a row with the player who is being chased at the other end. They start to chase each other.

2   The caller must work to protect the player who is being chased. She does this by giving a signal to the rows of players. When she calls out 'alleys!', the players making the rows drop their hands, turn to the right and join hands with their new neighbours. The new rows they make are the 'alleys'.

3   The caller must try to time her signal so that the player being chased is protected by the change in direction of play.

4   The chaser continues to chase until he has caught the other player or gives up.

Suggestion

The chaser and chased must keep to the streets and alleys: they must not duck underneath players' arms nor hold on to the players in the rows.

Adapting to others

9 Games with rules

Rules in games dictate how much time players have to do something, how they move in a game, where they move to, where they are safe and where there is danger. Rules concern how players are tagged or captured and how they are freed. There can also be rules about who is 'It' and what player is in which team. Traditional games tend to be more rule based than newer games and some have rules that are these days cast in a questionable light. Traditional games may involve running away from a player whose touch is 'poison', for example, or taunting others and ganging up as part of the game. This can be problematic for some children including some children with autism. Children with autism have difficulty distinguishing real from pretend and may not be able to see the difference between playful and actual teasing.

The point about playing games with rules is here seen as an opportunity for children to experience the challenges involved. Challenge lies in the richness and complexity of the games, the amount of coordination required between players, and the sophistication of the play. For children with autism, in particular, challenge lies too in the amount of flexibility needed to play these games. Players must cope not only with rules that change, but also with having to sort out the frequent disputes that arise in games with rules. Playing games with rules may not be right for all children, but can be very rewarding for some.

Key terms

rule, changing the rule, sorting out differences, for the sake of the game

Rules used

- guessing the rule of the game
- playing within a time limit
- moving in a special way
- finding an area that is 'safe'
- another player becoming 'It'
- having a 'danger zone'
- having players who are 'friends' and others who are 'enemies'
- having to perform a special task
- having special rituals for catching and freeing players
- players changing sides.

The Rule of the Game

One player guesses the rule that the rest of the group have secretly agreed to.

Organisation of players

One player volunteers to be the guesser. The rest of the group must abide by the rule without giving it away.

Playing the game

1 The player who is the guesser leaves the group.

2 The group discuss what the rule should be. For example, the rule might be that when players answer a question, they must cross their legs, or answer as if they were the person sitting on their right, or say 'Umm' before they speak.

3 When the group is ready, the guesser returns.

4 The guesser asks players questions which they must answer using the rule of the game.

5 The guesser has two or more chances to guess what the rule is.

Suggestion

This game is useful for conveying the idea not only that games have rules, but that there can be different rules and that they are changeable. An alternative way of playing the game is for players to carry out a mime according to the rule. Instead of questioning players, the guesser asks them to perform an action.

Name Six

In this circle game, players must name six items within a set time.

Organisation of players

Players stand in a circle. One player, who is the caller, stands outside the circle. Players need one ball or beanbag.

Playing the game

1   The ball is passed around the circle.

2   The caller, standing outside the circle in a place where he can see all the players, calls out a letter of the alphabet.

3   When the letter is called, the player holding the ball must name six items beginning with that letter. For example, if the letter is 'B', the player answers 'Bottle, bag, bicycle, bin, bed, bench'.

4   Before he gives the six items he quickly passes on the ball to start the time he has to name them.

5   The ball is passed around the circle. The player must say his six items before the ball reaches him again.

6   When his turn is finished, the ball is passed again until the caller says another letter of the alphabet.

Suggestion

To adjust the difficulty of the game, players can be asked to name, say, three or ten items.

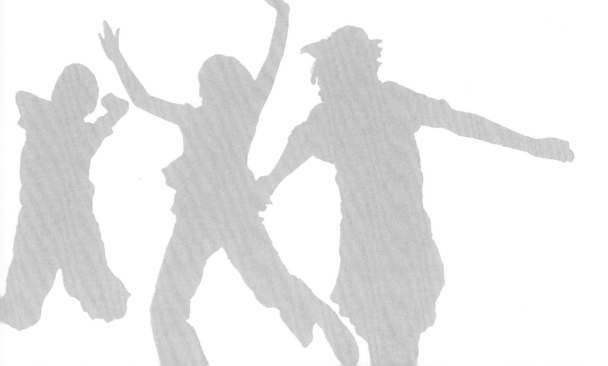

Move Like Spidey

Players must correctly guess information about an object to be able to move forward in the game.

Organisation of players

Players decide which character in Spiderman they are going to be, for example, Spiderman, Mary Jane, Aunt May, Dr Octopus, the Green Goblin. It does not matter if some players choose to be the same character. Players line up as a starting point. One player volunteers to think of an object and stands a distance away facing the line of players.

Playing the game

1   The players who are lined up take turns to ask questions about the object, to which the player can only answer 'yes' or 'no'.

2   If they get a correct answer they can move forward one step towards the player who is answering the questions. They must move in the style of their character, which must be established before the game begins. For example, Spiderman jumps, Mary Jane walks bravely, Aunt May takes small nervous steps, Green Goblin glides on his hoverboard, and so on.

3   When a player reaches the other side, he becomes the player who thinks of an object and the game begins again.

Suggestion

The fun in this game is in the movement of the players. Do not let the thinking up or guessing of an object become a sticking point for the whole game. If some children have difficulty guessing or thinking of an object, use a selection of photographs of objects at the beginning of the game. These give ideas for players to surreptitiously choose as well as limiting possibilities in terms of the guessing.

An advantage of this game is that any set of characters can be used, perhaps those from a favourite film or television programme.

Think About!

'For the sake of the game'

Games with rules have an advantage in terms of clarity of purpose, but the disadvantage is that they lead to more disputes among players. In playing games, children most frequently argue about taking on disliked roles and about whether someone is abiding by a rule. The games that follow are fast paced, with a high chance of disputes arising between players.

It should be remembered that conflict in play, and indeed in friendship, is completely natural. Children who are friends are involved in more conflict than those who are not. Getting into arguments, falling out and sorting out differences are all part of everyday social interaction, and conflict should not be seen as something that is wrong or naughty. What is important is to help children manage their conflicts.

Fortunately, children have their own ways of managing conflict which they can be encouraged to use. A very important consideration for children is that they should be able to keep playing a game for as long as possible. Players can entreat others to sort out their differences 'for the sake of the game', to sort out, make up or give in so that the game can go on. Disputes can also be decided using chance, dipping to see who should be 'It' or whose argument should prevail. It is also possible to allow players to decide how they want to carry out a disliked role, for example, to choose to be a more powerful 'It'.

Children think about:

When we disagree about the rules of a game we can:

- argue – it is natural to argue and everyone has arguments.
  It is important not to have too many arguments or let them go on for too long
- change the rule or the game – the games we play are adaptable.
  This means that we are allowed to change the game or the rule to suit ourselves
- dip – if two players disagree about something we can try dipping and leave the decision to chance
- start again – we can play the game again.

Little Packets

There are many versions of this traditional game, where one child chases another around a line of players.

Organisation of players

Players make lines of three, standing one behind the other and all facing in the same direction. Lines of players can be parallel to each other or form a shape, such as a cross, but they should not be joined. One player is the chaser and another is chased.

Playing the game

1   The chaser and chased run around the 'packets' formed by the other players, one trying to catch the other.

2   The player who is being chased can 'find safety' and opt out of the chase at any point by joining one end of a packet.

3   When he does so, the player who is at the other end of the line must become 'It'.

4   She leaves the line and must run away from the chaser. However, she too can choose to opt out at any point, by joining a line.

5   A line must never have more than three players in a packet.

6   If the chaser catches the other player, they swap roles or two new players are chosen.

Suggestion

Many chase games can be done at a different pace. If running makes the game too fast, players can decide that they must walk or move in some other prescribed way.

Cat and Mouse

This is an exciting chase game with players frequently changing their role.

Organisation of players

Players are in pairs, holding hands. One player, the mouse, is being chased and another, the cat, is the chaser.

Playing the game

1   The players holding hands walk around the play space.

2   The cat chases the mouse around the players.

3   The mouse can find safety by joining a group of players, holding hands and making a group of three.

4   When he does so, the player on the other side of him must leave the group.

5   She is now the cat and the player who was chasing is transformed into the mouse.

6   They continue the chase, with the new mouse able to find safety in the same way.

Suggestion

Sometimes the new mouse needs a little time to get away. In a variation of the game, the cat counts to ten before beginning the chase again.

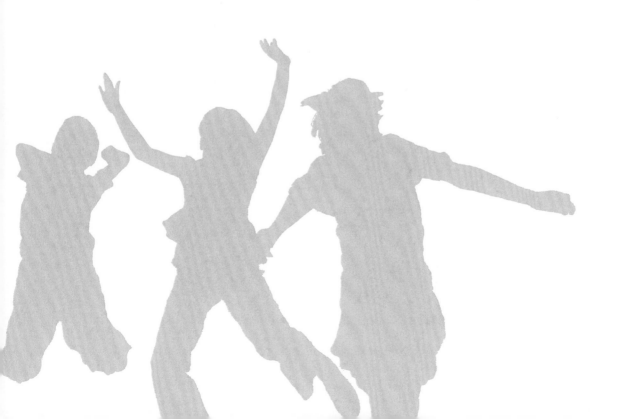

Jack's Ground

This game introduces the idea that part of the play space is dangerous or toxic in some way.

Organisation of players

A large circle is drawn on the ground in chalk as a danger zone. One player is 'It' and stands in 'Jack's ground', the danger zone. All the other players line up on the edges of the danger zone.

Playing the game

1 Players around the edge must go into the danger zone without being tagged.

2 They can taunt the player who is 'It' by stepping inside and calling out:

   Here I am, hanging round,

   All day long, in Jack's ground.

3 The player who is 'It' must try to tag players who come inside the danger zone.

4 Players who are tagged change sides and help with the catching.

Suggestion

The danger zone does not have to be designated as 'Jack's ground'. The child who is 'It' can pretend to be a zombie, vampire or dangerous animal and can be in 'the zombie pit', 'the graveyard' or 'the jungle'. The taunting can be rephrased accordingly.

Bomb and Shield

Playing this game several times ensures different players are chosen to be bomb and shield.

Organisation of players

Players move freely around the play area. One player is the caller.

Playing the game

1   As the players walk around the space, they choose two other children in the group; one is a 'bomb' and the other is their 'shield'. This is done without telling players what role they have.

2   Once they have chosen, players must get themselves into the position where their 'shield' is between them and their 'bomb'. This will involve children dodging around the play space, no one knowing who is what.

3   After a few minutes, the caller begins a countdown to the explosion of the bomb.

Suggestion

This game can be played as a 'friend' and 'enemy' game by telling players that they must get as far away from their enemy as they can, who they try not to look at or speak to, and close to their friend, who they can smile at and say hello to.

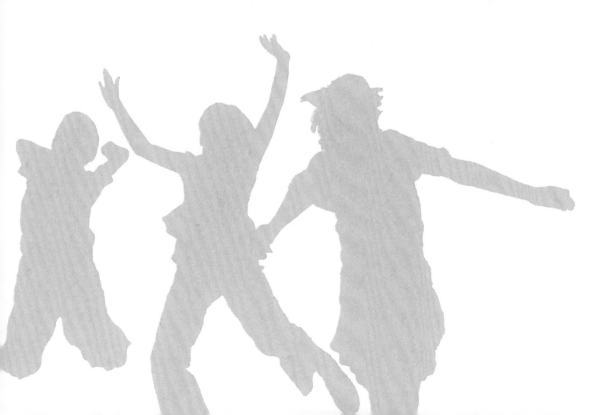

Whip

This game involves players having to perform a special task in order to reach 'home'.

Organisation of players

An area of the play space is established as 'home'. One player is the seeker, the other players hide.

Playing the game

1   The seeker closes her eyes and counts to twenty while the players find a hiding place.

2   When the seeker is finished counting, she looks for the players.

3   When she sees a player, she calls out their name and they stand up in full view, staying where they are.

4   The seeker continues to look for players until all the players are found.

5   When all the players have been found, they take it in turns to get home.

6   The seeker estimates the number of steps a player will take to reach the area that is 'home'. Steps can be pigeon steps (small steps, toes turned in), baby crawl (crawl on the ground), star jumps, bunny hops, giant strides, and so on.

7   For each player, the seeker says how many of a certain step the player will need to take to reach home.

8   The player then takes that number of steps. If they reach home in that time they are safe; if not, they must become the next seeker.

Suggestion

This game does not rely on children being good at hiding. The fun to be had is in the getting home.

Relievo

This is a sophisticated game of hide-and-seek with a den, a danger area and special rituals for getting caught and being freed.

Organisation of players

Players must mark out the various areas of the game before the start. In the centre of the play space there should be a 'den', essentially a holding pen, which is marked out visually with chalk. Around this den, a larger danger zone is marked out.

Players divide into two teams. Each team chooses a 'den warden' who stands beside the den.

Playing the game

1   The players in Team A stand inside the den and close their eyes while the players in Team B run away and hide.

2   When they are hidden, their den warden calls out 'Ready!' Team A players open their eyes and fan out, searching for players in Team B.

3   When a hider is seen, he is 'caught' in a special way with the seeker putting a hand on his shoulder and saying 'Two, four, six, eight, ten'. A hider can avoid capture by running away before the count is finished.

4   When a player is caught, he is formally marched to the den and guarded by Team A's den warden.

5   Team B's prisoners can be freed by a player from their side. The player must sneak through the danger zone without the den warden seeing them, step into the den area and shout 'Relievo!'. This is the signal for all prisoners to escape. The den warden can catch them if he tags them in the danger zone, but outside of that they become free.

6   When all players in one team have been captured or when the team that is seeking gives up, the players swap their roles and the game begins again.

Suggestion

The den warden is a strenuous role and can be shared by two or three players.

Red Rover

This is a strenuous game which can be exhilarating for children to play.

Organisation of players

Players divide into two teams. Each team selects a leader. Teams line up facing each other 15 metres apart.

Playing the game

1   Players hold hands.

2   One team begins with the leader calling out the name of a player in the opposite team, saying 'Red Rover, Red Rover, we call Sara over!' (naming the player).

3   The player who has been named must try to break through the line of the opposing team. She charges at the line, trying to break the grip of two players who are holding hands.

4   If she succeeds, she returns to her side, bringing an opposing player with her. If she does not manage to break through, she must stay with that team, changing sides.

5   The game begins again, with the caller from the second team naming an opposing player.

Suggestion

These days, games such as Red Rover are often deemed too dangerous for children to play. However, like Bull in the Ring, when played well it can prove to be a very satisfying experience of physical exertion.

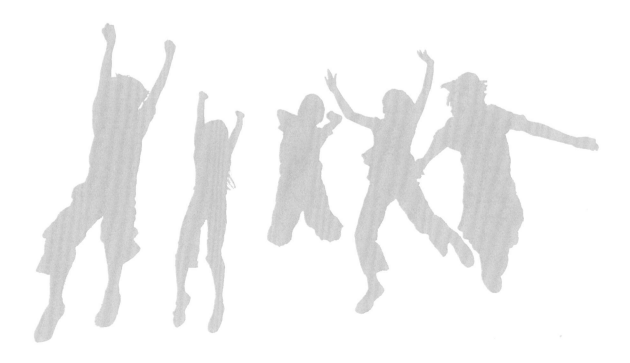

Creativity

We know that children with autism are able to perform pretend acts and generate imaginative ideas. What is hard, however, is the social aspect of play, the coordinated responses of two or more children, combining play elements and building on each other's ideas to create an elaborate play world.

The games that follow involve playing together in a way that is more creative, inventive and collaborative. An important aspect of children's traditional games is that they have variation and are open to adaptation by the players. The games here pick up on this element, encouraging children to generate their own ideas within a game, to add their own expressions and actions, to create narratives and invent games of their own.

Traditional games are influenced by the general culture, so that recent events and popular culture determine the details of games and the characters involved. Children also traditionally use their own lives and personal interests as material for playing games. Children with autism are often very interested in certain aspects of popular culture and may have strong personal interests about which they have a good deal of knowledge. Both these facts can be usefully employed when encouraging creativity in children and thinking up new versions of a game.

Creativity

10 Games of expression

Being creative in play involves carrying out pretend actions, putting on voices, using the body expressively, adopting roles, improvising actions and inventing dialogue and stories. Playing often involves a sophisticated combination of a number of these elements, making it hard for some children, particularly children with autism, to access play. It is possible, however, to introduce children to activities and games that call on only one or two of these skills and that are therefore more inclusive.

The next games concern expression only, the expressive use of the body, face and hands. There is very little here in the way of improvising. Some games require players to speak lines, but these are already given as part of the game. The games are designed to encourage children to move – move their face and body, get their muscles working – and have fun with being physically expressive. They are also encouraged to watch other children's expressions and learn from them. The first four games involve very simple individual expressive poses, using characters with a strong appeal to children. Two games that involve action songs are given as a way of practising moving expressively. The final games concern carrying out simple pretend actions within a group, coordinating pretence with other children.

Key terms

face, hands and body, moving, watching others

Progression of skills

• adopt an expressive pose

• move with expression

• be expressive as part of a group.

Wizards, Giants and Elves

This game requires players to adopt the correct pose for three different characters.

Organisation of players

One player is nominated as the caller. The remaining players divide into two teams.
Teams organise themselves as equally as possible into three groups of wizards, giants and elves.
When both teams are ready, they stand in a line, the players at the front facing each other.

Playing the game

1   The caller shouts out 'One, two, three, go!' and the first players in each line stand forward in character, revealing who they are. Wizards should adopt a pose brandishing a magic wand, giants act is if they are huge, marching forward and roaring, elves crouch down and look nervous.

2   One player beats the other by virtue of their character:

   Wizards beat giants by casting a spell on them.

   Giants beat elves by stamping on them.

   Elves beat wizards by running up their cloak and strangling them.

3   It is important that both players reveal their characters at the same time. The caller decides this and sends players back to begin again if necessary.

4   The game continues with all players in the line revealing themselves.

Suggestion

Any combination of characters can be used for this game. A variation that is highly enjoyable is 'Dr Who', with the Doctor standing forward holding his sonic screwdriver, a dalek with a raised arm as a mechanical eyestick, and a Cyberman who marches forward. Children can decide who beats whom.

Dracula

The more expression a player puts in to being Dracula, the more fun it is to play the game.

Organisation of players

One player is Dracula and adopts a suitably threatening pose. All the other players are his victims. They move freely about but must try to avoid making eye contact with Dracula.

Playing the game

1   Dracula finds a victim by catching someone's eye.

2   As soon as he 'hooks' a victim in this way, he starts to walk menacingly towards the player. That player must stand still as Dracula approaches.

3   The threatened player must try catch the eye of another player, who calls out her name to release her from Dracula's power. If she is released, the game continues with Dracula looking for another victim.

4   If the player is not released, Dracula can pretend to bite her neck.

Suggestion

Maintaining eye contact can be an issue for some children with autism, although the fun to be had playing this game usually minimises that difficulty.

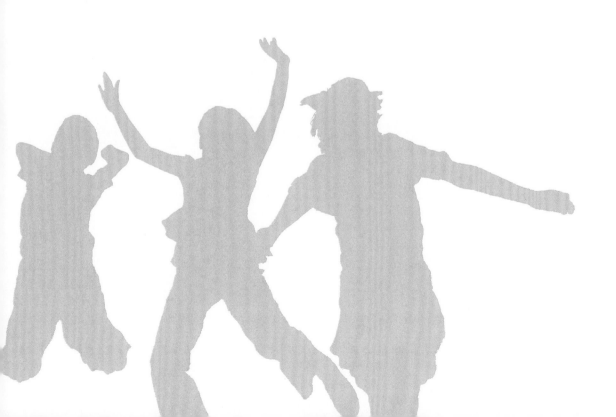

Superhero Initials

This is a game for boys in particular to enjoy.

Organisation of players

One player decides what superhero pose they will adopt and thinks of a phrase or sentence typically associated with that character.

Playing the game

1   When the player is ready, he steps towards the other players in role, adopting the pose of that character.

2   The other players begin to guess which superhero he is.

3   They can ask 'What is your name?', to which the player should reply in role, giving the initials only. For example, if he is Iron Man, he should say 'My name is I. M.'

4   Players then ask 'What do you say?', to which the player in role replies, giving the typical phrase or sentence associated with that character.

5   Players try to guess who the superhero is.

Suggestion

To help children get into character, it is possible to look through magazines and books or even on the internet before playing the game.

Queenie, Queenie, Who's Got the Ball?

This is traditionally a game that girls play, although all children can enjoy it.

Organisation of players

One player is nominated to be Queen and stands with her back to the other players. Players form a long line.

Playing the game

1 With the players lined up, Queenie throws a ball behind her without looking around.

2 One player catches the ball and hides it as best he can. All the other players put their hands behind their backs.

3 The players tell Queenie they are ready by chanting:

   Queenie, Queenie, who's got the ball

   Is she big or is she small

   Queenie, Queenie, who's got the ball?

4 Queenie turns round and, adopting a regal pose, begins to inspect the line of players.

5 She asks a player in a queenly voice, 'Have you got the ball?'.

6 If she guesses correctly, she remains Queenie and the game begins again. If she chooses a player incorrectly, that player becomes queen.

Suggestion

More fun can be had if Queenie asks players to do certain things, such as stretch out an arm, shake a leg, jump up and down or bend over.

Think About!

Watching and doing

Although some children with autism have difficulty maintaining eye contact with another person, watching others is often an important way for them to learn about social interaction and communication. Watching others is not a passive act but an active taking in of social experience. For all individuals, watching the actions and expressions of others is a way of knowing about and being able to do something. For individuals with autism in particular, it is a social activity that is perhaps more accessible than direct face-to-face interaction and discussion. Children should be put into situations where they can watch the social engagement of others, including others playing games and singing songs. Standing in a circle is a good way of being able to observe the actions of others.

Watching other people's expressions is also important, given that many children with autism have poor proprioception and may not get effective muscular feedback from their own body, face and hands. By watching themselves in the mirror, pulling their face into different expressions with their hands, and watching others, they can learn to be more expressive.

Children think about:

I can teach my body to be expressive by:

• watching others – looking at what they do with their faces to show different feelings, what they do with their hands and how they move their bodies

• looking in the mirror – to see what my face looks like when I try to make different expressions

• trying to be aware of my own body, as if I can see myself in a mirror – trying to be aware of my face and what it is doing, of my hands and how I am standing.

Jelly on a Plate

Children can have fun with the actions in this well-known singing game.

Organisation of players
Children stand round in a circle or simply stand together in a group.

Playing the game
Children sing the choruses of the song while acting out the actions that accompany it:

> *Jelly on a plate, jelly on a plate*
> *Wibble-wobble, wibble-wobble* [Make a wobbling action]
> *Jelly on a plate*
>
> *Sausage in a pan, sausage in a pan*
> *Turn it over, turn it over* [Turn around twice]
> *Sausage in a pan*
>
> *Baby on the floor, baby on the floor*
> *Pick it up, pick it up* [Picking up action]
> *Baby on the floor*
>
> *Burglar in the house, burglar in the house*
> *Kick him out, kick him out* [Kicking action]
> *Burglar in the house*

Suggestion
Teach children other songs with actions and sing them together.

The Little Green Frog

This is a very funny song that makes children laugh.

Organisation of players

Children stand round in a circle or simply stand together in a group.

Playing the game

Children sing the two choruses of this song in two different expressive styles. The first chorus is sung in a rude and rough fashion, the second more sedately and slowly, except for the last bit:

Mmm-uh [sticking out tongue on 'uh'] *said the little green frog one day*

Mmm-uh [sticking out tongue on 'uh'] *said the little green frog*

Mmm-uh [sticking out tongue on 'uh'] *said the little green frog one day*

And the little green frog said Mmm-uh-ahhh

[sticking out tongue on 'uh', shaking head and hands on 'ahhh']

Buuuuut, we know that frogs go

Mmm-la-di-da-di-da [making sedate walking movements]

Mmm-la-di-da-di-da [making sedate walking movements]

Mmm-la-di-da-di-da [making sedate walking movements]

We know that frogs go

Mmm-la-di-da-di-da [making sedate walking movements]

They don't go

Mmm-uh-ahhh

[sticking out tongue on 'uh', shaking head and hands on 'ahhh']

Suggestion

Any two tunes will work with this song, as long as the second is slower and 'posher' than the first.

Driving

Players work in pairs for this game.

Organisation of players

Players organise themselves into pairs. One of the players is a car and the other is the driver. The driver lines up behind his car, both car and driver facing in the same direction.

Playing the game

1 Explain to the children how they drive their car using special signals communicated through touch. To drive the car, drivers simply rest their hand on the centre of the back of the player who is the car. To make the following manoeuvres, they use these signals:

> To turn left – touch on the left shoulder
>
> To turn right – touch on the right shoulder
>
> Stop – hand taps the centre of the back

2 Drivers begin to drive their car around the play space. They should take care to drive responsibly, avoiding bumping into anything or hitting another vehicle.

3 Players swap roles and play the game again.

Suggestion

The idea of controlling another person using special signals appeals to most children. Encourage them to invent other signals, using more touch signals.

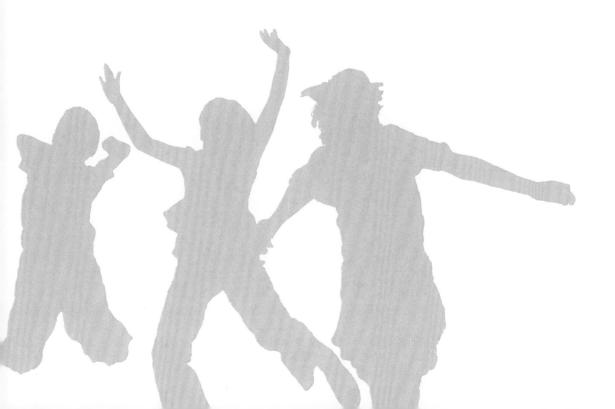

Adverb Game

Children carry out individual actions, but do so altogether as part of a group.

Organisation of players

One player volunteers to be the guesser and moves away from the play space, standing at a distance or going out of the room.

Playing the game

1   The group decides together on an adverb to use for the game, such as 'slowly', 'kindly', sadly' or 'excitedly'.

2   The player who is the guesser returns and instructs the whole group to perform actions which must be done according to the agreed adverb. For example, the guesser says 'Wave goodbye that way' or, 'Ask for some sweets that way'.

3   The group perform each action in turn, each player doing the action at the same time as the rest of the group.

4   The guesser tries to guess the adverb.

5   Actions continue until she guesses correctly or gives up.

Suggestion

Another way to play the game is for the group to think up actions themselves, or simply to walk around in the style of the adverb.

Construction Site

This is a game of group invention.

Organisation of players

Players organise themselves into smaller groups of two to six members. They find a space which is their construction site.

Playing the game

1   Players think of a structure to build. Examples of structures would be a suspension bridge, a skyscraper, a car, a dome or a house.

2   Groups are given time to plan, design and build their structure. Structures are made by players using their hands, arms, legs and bodies. They may also use whatever objects are to hand, such as jumpers and bags.

3   Groups take it in turn to show each other their construction.

Suggestion

Anything can be made in this way. Children can make natural phenomena, such as trees or clouds, or they can make letters and numbers, or they can make rooms of the school, all for other players to guess what they are.

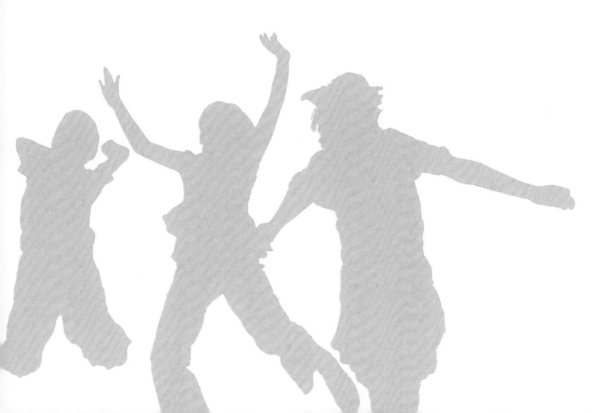

Adverts

This game requires imagination and creativity.

Organisation of players

Players take it in turn, or work in twos or threes, to create a living advert.

Playing the game

1   Individual players or small groups spend some time planning the advert. They decide what it is they are advertising and how they are going to do it. Adverts can be for anything, including books, films, toys or even the players themselves.

2   An advert should consist of two things: a 'picture' which is made by the players freezing in a certain pose or scene, and a line about their product, which is spoken by the players.

3   Players take turns to show their adverts to the rest of the group.

4   The group say what they think is being advertised.

Suggestion

It does help to remind children of what an advert looks like, either by recalling familiar adverts to mind or by looking through magazines and finding good examples to copy.

Creativity

11 Games with stories

Children with autism often have difficulty making up a story, but stories do not have to be entirely new to be used in play. In fact, all children base their stories on familiar themes, using a similar structure of events each time. Games that involve making up stories often have a built-in structure for children to follow to help with the creation of a story.

The games here provide structure in different ways, beginning with simple story making and developing towards the creation of more sophisticated stories. The first three games are fun to play but at the same time provide players with a simple story structure. The next games focus on peers supporting each other in their storytelling. Naturally, in children's play, more experienced players help to keep a game going by providing more input than less experienced, often younger, players. This idea is used here in four games that concern making up stories in pairs where one player may be relied on to do more work than their partner. The final three games provide basic story ideas only, leaving it open for children to expand on a theme. However, the 'Think About' discussion provides the most frequent story routines found in children's play, which can be shared with players as a basis for their story making.

Key terms
and then, action, feeling

Progression of skills
- make up a story using a given structure
- make up a story in a pair
- make up a new story using familiar elements.

One-Word Stories

This is a very simple way of creating a story in a group.

Organisation of players

Children sit in a circle or in a line.

Playing the game

1   One player starts by saying a word. Alternatively, all stories can start with the first four players saying 'Once – upon – a – time – ', the story carrying on from there.

2   Going around the circle or along the line, each player contributes one word only to the story.

3   The story goes round the players until it comes to a natural end, usually the end of a sentence.

4   It works well to use the names of the children themselves in the story so that funny one-word stories are made up about them.

Suggestion

The stories that are made in this way can be very strange indeed, although they are often quite funny. It works well if more able children sit between less able or younger ones. This helps to ensure that stories 'flow' and do not become too crazy!

One-Prop Stories

In this game, the use of a prop provides ideas for how a story should develop.

Organisation of players

Children sit in a group. They have one prop between them.

Playing the game

1   The first player who can think of a beginning to a story starts. In giving an opening sentence, he must include the use of the prop. The prop can be used to represent any object that it reasonably resembles. For example, a prop such as a chopstick can become a wand, a sword, a ladder or a match.

2   Players take it in turns to contribute to the story, thinking up the next part. They must include the prop each time.

3   The final player should try to end the story in some way.

Suggestion

Encourage players to think of new ways to transform the prop, but do not insist on it.
Some props are hard to transform into different objects. Do not worry if children use a prop in the same way as another player. Simple props with distinct shapes are the best to use and the easiest to transform, for example round, square or long objects, boxes and balls. Props can stand for anything that is big, medium or small in size as long as it is a similar shape.

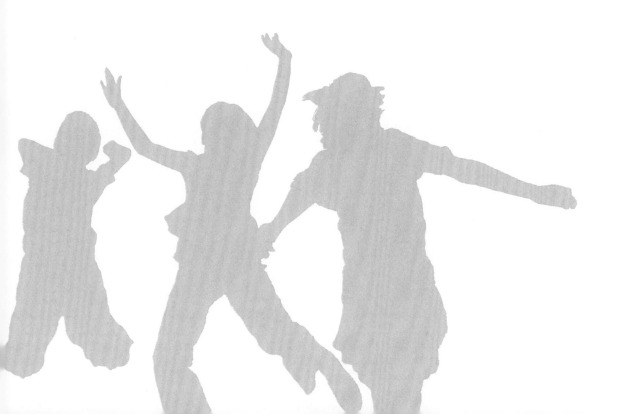

Prison Breakout

In this game, children embellish a prison escape story.

Organisation of players

Players are in groups of three or four.

Playing the game

1   Each player in a group is asked to choose a household object.

2   The group is given the following instruction: 'You are in prison and you must try to break out. To escape you have to climb over a wall, then get over a barbed-wire fence. You then have to cross a piranha-infested river and finally go through an impenetrable jungle. After that, you will be free. All you have to help you is the household objects you have chosen. Good luck.'

3   The group discuss quickly how they are going to use their household objects to help in the escape.

4   They carry out the prison break by acting out their escape using their imaginary props. One child in a group – or all the children together – can narrate the story of the breakout as it is being acted out.

Suggestion

Some children might prefer to pretend using real props, in which case a box of ordinary objects can be used for players to choose from. Similarly, some groups may find pretending easier if they are climbing over and going through real objects, such as over low walls or benches and across grass or a playground.

Two Rush In

In this game, two players support each other in improvising a story.

Organisation of players

In pairs, children take it in turn to do this activity while the rest of the group listen to their story.

Playing the game

1   The group sit together except for one pair who stand to one side.

2   The pair rush towards the group in an excited way.

3   They begin to tell a story about something extraordinary that has just happened.

4   The two players take it in turns to tell the story, for example, 'We were just going out to play' – 'and we saw this amazing spaceship fly over the school' – 'and then it landed in the playground' – 'and do you know who came out?' – and so on.

5   One player must try to follow on from what the other player has said in the story.

Suggestion

This game works well if a little thought is given to who to partner with whom. The idea of peer-supported stories is that one peer is helping the other to generate a story, but taking it in turns also means that one player does not dominate the game.

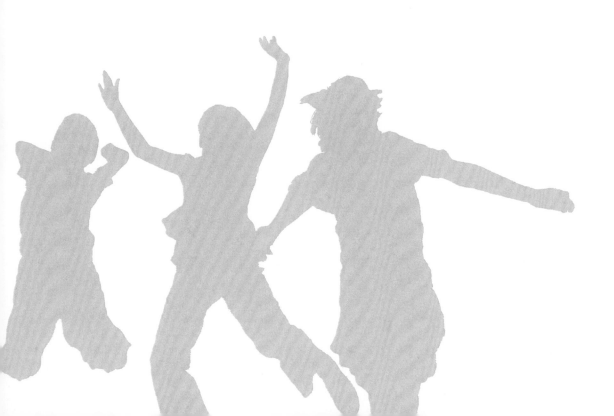

Hey, You!

One player must create an excuse for having something that belongs to another player.

Organisation of players

The group stand in a circle with one player in the middle. Various everyday objects are to hand, for example, a jumper, a bag or a book.

Playing the game

1   The player in the middle of the circle chooses one object to use for the game and gives it to a player in the circle. She closes her eyes.

2   The object is passed around the circle.

3   When the player in the middle claps her hands, whoever has been passed the object must hold on to it.

4   The player in the middle opens her eyes and looks round the circle accusingly, to see who has 'her object'. She says 'Hey, you, why have you got my ___?'

5   The player who has the item must make up an excuse for why they have something that belongs to someone else. He can provide as elaborate a story as he wants.

6   The player in the middle interrogates him by asking questions.

7   The player who has the object eventually apologises and gives back the item, or the player in the middle, if she likes his story, can tell him to keep it.

Suggestion

This game can be played as an improvisation if the two players put more feeling into their roles of accuser and excuser, the first being angry and the second nervous.

Embellishing Stories

One player is used to expand on the story of another.

Organisation of players

In pairs, children find somewhere comfortable to sit.

Playing the game

1   One child thinks of a story to tell his partner. The story can be about something that has happened to him recently or can be based on a book or a film.

2   He tells the story in a simple way, breaking it into sections. After each section, he pauses.

3   When he pauses, his partner tells that bit of the story back to him. She must try to add as much as embellishment to the story as possible, without actually changing the details of the story.

Suggestion

Think carefully about who to partner with whom and do not expect partners necessarily to swap roles. Adding detail to a story requires some skill and may be something that only some children are able to do.

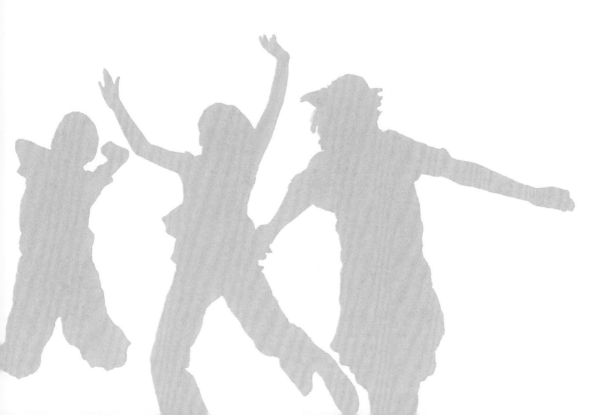

Star Wars

Children need to be familiar with the film Star Wars to play this game, but any familiar book or TV programme can be used.

Organisation of players

The group form pairs. Each pair chooses two characters from Star Wars and decides who is going to play which part. They decide on a scene from the film which involves these two characters.

Playing the game

1   In pairs, children act out their chosen scene. One partner describes what the other character does, and the other partner then acts this out. For example, player A says 'Luke Skywalker jumped into his landspeeder' and player B then acts this out.

2   The second player then does the same, telling the next bit of the action concerning player A's character. For example, player B says 'The stormtrooper shoots at Skywalker with his blaster rifle' and player A acts this out.

3   The story is continued in this way, each player being responsible for the action done by his partner.

4   Players can also give instructions about the lines a character must speak.

Suggestion

If it is too difficult for both players to tell the story, it is possible for one partner to be responsible for the storytelling with the pair taking it in turns to act out their respective parts.

Think About!

Story routines

Children's imaginative play often appears to be complex and elaborate, but actually revisits familiar themes and often repeats the same underlying story routines. Children with autism can be introduced to some of these routines so that they are better able to understand what is happening in pretend play. The most popular story routines in children's play are provided below. The highlighted elements, which include appropriate emotions, can be included in a visual storyboard for children to follow.

Children think about:

Lost and found
- Something is **hidden**
- You **realise** this and **worry**
- You **search** for it
- You **discover** it and are **happy**

Danger
- You are on the **lookout** for danger
- You **see** danger
- You take **evasive action**
- You are **relieved** – the danger has gone

Monsters
- One person is **recognised as a threat**, (eg a monster, zombie or dangerous animal)
- They walk around and everyone **runs away** from them, trying to hide or keep out of the way
- It is both **exciting** and **frightening**

Fighting
- There are **two sides**
- Each has a **distinguishing feature** and a **special ability**
- There is a **fight** sequence – with no real touching, only movement and noise

Families
- You are **humans** or **animals**
- You are a **family** or some other kind of community
- You **live** somewhere
- You **look after** each other and carry out ordinary daily activities

Acting Out a Film

Children can base their stories on the plot of a favourite film.

Organisation of players

Children play in small groups, with enough players for the number of characters in the film they are going to act out.

Playing the game

1   In their small groups, players decide on what film they want to act out and choose three or four scenes from the film.

2   Players work out how they are going to act out each scene. They decide each player's character, where players stand at the beginning of the scene, what action takes place and what lines each character says.

3   Still in their small groups, players practise their scenes.

4   Once groups are happy with their 'film', they take it in turns to show it to the whole group, moving between each scene they have created.

Suggestion

Instead of acting out a film, groups can act out something that has happened to one of their members, a funny recent incident, a real-life dramatic event or something that happened when they were a baby.

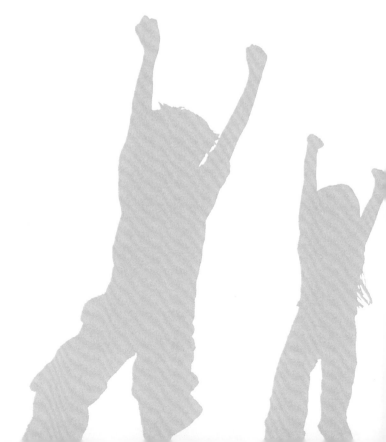

Favourite Stories

This is a way for children to share their enjoyment of favourite books and characters.

Organisation of players

Children play in small groups with one player being the narrator.

Playing the game

1   In their group, players decide what characters are in their story. They agree what a character typically does and says. For example, if the group decide to use *Charlie and the Chocolate Factory* as their story, they may decide that Charlie smiles and looks nice, Augustus Gloop eats messily, Veruca Salt walks around in a posh way, Violet Beauregarde does sporty moves and Mike Teevee looks angry and aggressive, punching the air.

2   The narrator then tells the story. As a character is mentioned, the player steps forward and performs his character's action. If two characters are mentioned, both step forward in role.

Suggestion

The job of the narrator is a difficult one in this game and should be taken on by a child who is good at telling stories. Children can decide to tell only one part of a story, perhaps a particularly dramatic bit.

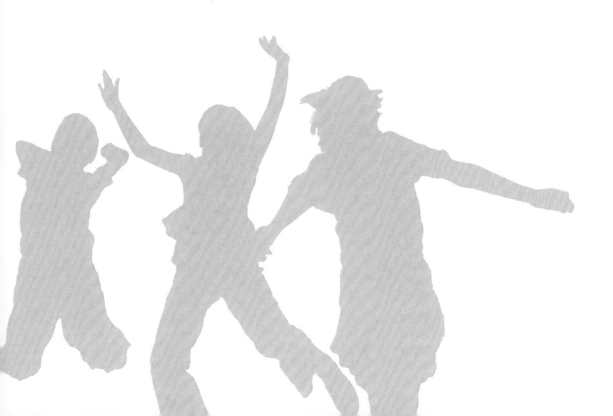

Wrong Stories

This game challenges children to tell a story that does not make sense.

Organisation of players

One player tells a story to the group.

Playing the game

1 The player who is going to tell the story thinks of a story or uses a known story. He can write out the story if he wishes.

2 He tells the story to the group. In telling the story, he inserts blatant errors, for example, 'Last summer, when it was snowing …' or 'For Christmas I got a cat that had three puppies …'.

3 The group listen carefully to the story, shouting out 'Wrong!' when they hear an error.

4 Alternatively, the players who are listening can work in twos or threes and write down an error as they hear it. At the end of the game, players can compare how many errors they noticed.

Suggestion

This game is similar to the idea of 'What's Wrong with this Picture?', but using listening instead of looking. The player who tells the story needs to be skilful and some children may only take part in the game as a listener. Alternatively, an adult can tell the story.

Creativity

12 Games of pretence

The following games involve players taking on a role and carrying out pretence in a coordinated way with other children. As a way of developing the capacity to do this, the games are organised into simple and more complex forms of improvisation. The first three games concern pretend sequences only, where the action and what the characters say to each other are prescribed within the game. The next three games are a little more open and require some improvisation on the part of the players. They concern short scenarios where two or more characters must improvise an interaction. Following this, there are three games that focus on improvising a scene, with structures for the improvisation built into each.

The final activity allows children to use what they know about games to invent some of their own. Encourage children to borrow ideas from their favourite games and incorporate their own interests and real-life experiences and routines. Allow children to take on roles in a game that are right for them and do not expect all children to play all parts. Above all, let the enjoyment of an activity be the guide in whatever games you play.

Key terms

real life, pretending, role play

Progression of skills

• pretend using a structured sequence

• pretend within a given scenario

• improvise a scene

• invent a new game.

Ghost in the Attic

This is a traditional game with a set sequence of actions.

Organisation of players

One player is the ghost and stands away from the other children in an area which is the attic. The other players stand together. One of them is the mother.

Playing the game

1   The mother sends each of her children in turn to the attic to fetch her blanket.

2   The eldest child is sent first. When he does not return, the second eldest is sent and so on until the youngest child is finally sent to fetch the blanket.

3   Each time a child goes to the attic, the ghost jumps out on him and says that he will be spirited away. The child is kept somewhere in the attic.

4   When no children are left, the mother herself goes to the attic.

5   The ghost jumps out on her but she stands up to him and demands to know what has happened to her children.

6   When she finds her children they all run away from the ghost.

Suggestion

Traditionally, this game is the antecedent to a chase, but can be enjoyed just as a simple game of pretend.

Fox and Chickens

This is a playlet with set lines for players to speak.

Organisation of players

One player is the fox, another is the hen and the remaining players her chicks. The chicks line up behind the hen, holding on to the waist of the player in front.

Playing the game

1   The fox crouches on the ground.

2   The hen, followed by her chicks, walks up to the fox.

3   The following dialogue is spoken:

> HEN: *What are you doing old fox?*
>
> FOX: *Picking up sticks.*
>
> HEN: *What for?*
>
> FOX: *To make a fire.*
>
> HEN: *What do you want a fire for?*
>
> FOX: *To cook a chicken.*
>
> HEN: *Where will you get a chicken?*
>
> FOX: *Out of your flock!*

4   At these words, the fox springs up and tries to catch the chick that is at the end of the line.

5   The hen must do her best to stop this from happening by swinging her line of chicks away from the fox.

6   When the fox catches a chick, he puts it in his den and the game begins again.

Suggestion

The game works better if an older and more able child, who can be wily and persistent, is chosen as the fox.

In the Cupboard

Many traditional children's games involve the ritual of being eaten.

Organisation of players

One player is a householder and another is a witch-type character. All the other players are different foods in the cupboard.

Playing the game

1   Players decide what food they are, for example, butter, milk, jam, burgers.

2   They sit together as if they were in a cupboard or refrigerator.

3   The witch, pretending to be friendly, comes to the door and knocks.

4   The householder answers, saying 'Yes, what do you want?'

5   The witch replies that she is hungry and wants some food.

6   The householder asks her what she wants to eat.

7   The witch begins to name different foods. If she guesses one of the players, the householder goes to fetch that player and gives him to the witch.

8   The witch takes home all the food she has guessed correctly and makes a meal from it.

Suggestion

In traditional versions of this game, the witch ritualistically eats the children after having cooked the food.

Can I Have My Game Back?

This scenario concerns a conflict, where one individual is angry and the other apologetic.

Organisation of players

Players stand higgledy-piggledy around the play space.

Playing the game

1   One player starts the pretence by going to another player and asking her to return the game she borrowed. He explains that he needs it straight away.

2   The second player is apologetic and says she will get it immediately.

3   This player has lent the game to another person. She goes to a third player and angrily demands the return of the game.

4   The third player has also lent out the game. He apologises and says he will return it as soon as he can. He goes to a fourth player and demands the game angrily.

5   The game continues – with the lender always demanding and angry and the borrower humble and apologetic – until all players have been approached.

Suggestion

The 'game' in question can be anything. It can be a board game, a computer programme, a DVD or a book. Let children decide this for themselves.

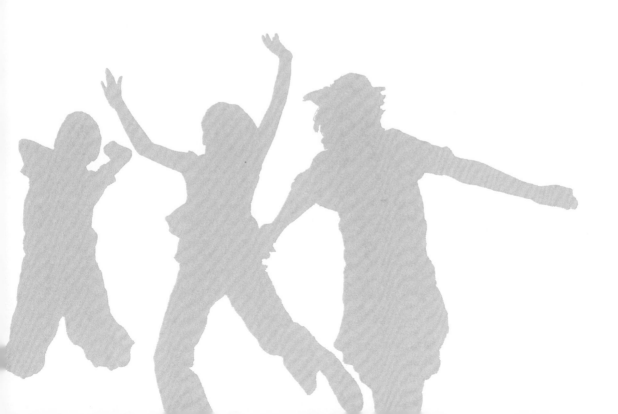

Choose your Punishment

Many children's games involve the idea of someone being punished, often a part of playing 'Schools'.

Organisation of players

One player is the questioner. Later in the scenario, this player becomes the authority figure in the scene.

Playing the game

1   The questioner asks each player what are the three punishments they most fear.

2   Players name their three punishments.

3   The players line up.

4   The questioner becomes the authority figure and, supported by two players as guards, he walks along the line selecting someone to be punished.

5   The authority figure can give a reason why the player is being punished or, on questioning, a player can admit to what it is she has done wrong.

6   When a player is selected she is taken from the line by the guards and receives one of her punishments.

7   The selection process continues.

Suggestion

Children who are not that dominant in the group may really enjoy taking on the very powerful authority figure role in this game.

Ask the Teacher

This is a funny game where children can have fun playing the teacher.

Organisation of players

One player is a pupil, another player is the teacher. The teacher decides on what kind of teacher she is, for example, kind and gentle, strict, dislikes children. The rest of the group watch the scene.

Playing the game

1 The two players enact a scene of teacher and pupil. The pupil either sits at his desk and raises his hand or goes up to the teacher's desk.

2 The pupil asks the teacher something, such as help or to go to the toilet.

3 The teacher responds to the request in role.

4 The players guess what kind of teacher she is.

Suggestion

In a funny version of this game, the teacher gradually transforms into something as she talks to the pupil, for example, the teacher gradually turns into an animal, growing ears, tail, teeth and so on. The other players must guess what the teacher has become. The teacher can turn into anything or anyone: a famous person, a magical character, a character from a book.

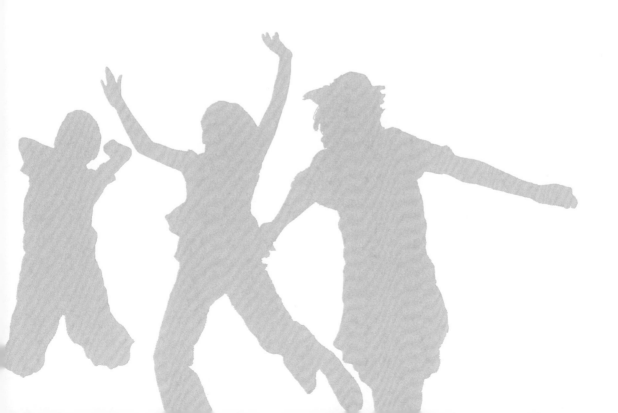

Voice-overs

Children create a voice-over for their favourite film or TV scenes. Video playback equipment is needed to play the game.

Organisation of players

Players need preparation time to watch their favourite scene from a film or TV programme. They should work in pairs or threes – enough players in a group to cover all the characters in the scene.

Playing the game

1   The players prepare by watching their chosen scene on replay. They may watch it as many times as they need. They may prepare a script or simply memorise the lines the characters in the scene say to each other.

2   When they are ready, they show the scene to the rest of the group. This involves the group watching the scene on a television or computer monitor with the volume turned down. The players, standing near the screen, provide the voice-over for the on-screen characters.

3   Groups take it in turn to listen to each other's voice-overs.

Suggestion

Some children may like to do the voice-overs for more than one character, adopting different voices for each one.

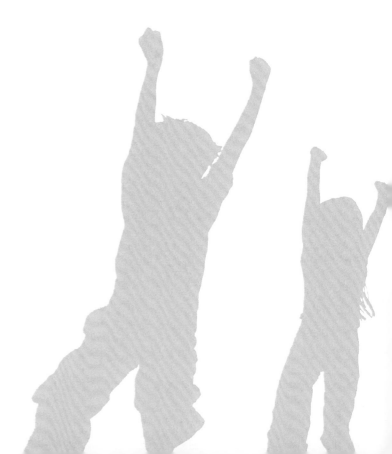

TV Interviews

Children can be interviewed as themselves or as a character they have chosen to be.

Organisation of players

One player is the TV host and interviewer. She has somewhere to sit and possibly a desk. Another chair is set out for the player who is the interviewee.

Playing the game

1 The TV host introduces the person she is about to interview, saying his name and what he is known for. The interviewee enters the scene.

2 The group watch and applaud as the interviewee enters.

3 The interview begins, the host asking questions and the interviewee responding.

4 Questions should be appropriate to whoever the interviewee is. If he is playing himself, he should be asked about his family, interests and personal history. If he is playing a character, he should be interviewed as that character.

5 Questions can also be asked by the 'live TV audience', that is, the players who are watching.

6 When the interview is over, the interviewee is thanked and applauded as he leaves.

Suggestion

Ensure that the child who is the interviewer has sufficient skill to bring out information from the other player. Alternatively, an adult can play the part of the interviewer.

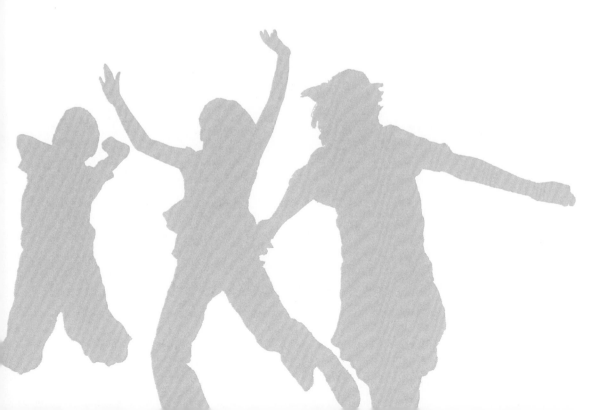

Congratulations

This game calls for sophisticated improvisation on the part of players to imply something without giving it away and to enquire without asking direct questions.

Organisation of players

One player volunteers to leave the room or move away from the play area.

Playing the game

1   The group agree on something imaginary that has just happened to this player.

2   The event must be something good for which congratulations are in order.

3   The player is called back to the group.

4   The group congratulates him without saying what it is he has done.

5   The player can play along with the scene, interacting and asking surreptitious questions to try to work out what it is that has happened to him.

6   When he thinks he knows, he guesses the reason for the congratulations.

Suggestion

The event might be something that is related to the real life, personality, abilities or interests of the player who is guessing.

Think About!

Inventing new games

Playing games is about invention, adapting familiar elements of games to suit the particular personalities, abilities and interests of the children playing. The worksheet below lists essential elements of games and can be used by children to support the invention of their own games.

Children think about:

What is the name of your game?

Does your game have someone who is 'It'?

Yes/No   If yes, how do you decide who is 'It'?

How are the players organised?

Pairs   Groups   Teams   Whole group

Are players a character or role?

Yes/No   If yes, what characters or roles?

How does the game start?

Eg delayed starter, suspense, one player as caller

Does your game have ...?

A hunt

A chase

Questions and answers

Magical or spooky elements

Action adventure

Is your game organised into different zones

Eg a den for prisoners, a safe haven, somewhere to run

What special skills must players have?

Being strong

Being fast

Being good at remembering (what?)

Being helpful or brave (what good does that do?)

Being able to make something (what?)

Special control over another/other players (how?)

Other

Does your game have a special word, line or song for players to say?

How does your game end?

Let's Play a Game!

Allow children to invent their own games.

Organisation of players

The group takes turns to play out each other's ideas.

Playing the game

1 The group are simply asked, 'Let's play a game. What game shall we play?'

2 Offer the possibility that children can make up their own game, using their knowledge and experience of other games.

3 Use the prompt sheet in the 'Think About' discussion to help children to invent their own game. Support the development of a game idea by asking probing questions.

4 Encourage children to bring their own interests, concerns and real-life experiences to their invented games.

Suggestion

Ensure that all children are heard in this process. Remember that games can be very short and very simple, consisting of only one or two elements.

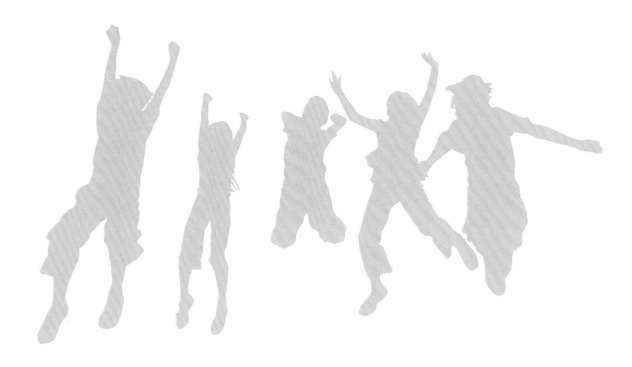

For Product Safety Concerns and Information please contact our EU
representative GPSR@taylorandfrancis.com Taylor & Francis Verlag GmbH,
Kaufingerstraße 24, 80331 München, Germany

Printed and bound by CPI Group (UK) Ltd, Croydon, CR0 4YY

01/05/2025

01858620-0001

PLAY BETTER GAMES

Carmel Conn

Ordinary games are an important vehicle for children's learning. They provide a powerful, naturally occurring learning environment that is physical, playful and fun. Playing games requires interpersonal skills in language, thought, social behavior, creativity, self-regulation and skilful use of the body. When children play games together they develop the following key capacities:

- Cooperative behavior
- Focused attention
- Social understanding
- Holding information in mind
- Motor, spatial and sequential planning
- Self-regulation, eg impulse control, coping with excitement, controlled exertion
- Collaborative behavior and negotiation
- Self-expression and creativity.

Games provide a social experience that is emotionally compelling, where children laugh and have fun and do not realise they are interacting, problem solving, negotiating and cooperating with each other.

Play Better Games is designed to help practitioners and parents to think about what might prohibit their children from joining in with games and plan effective strategies for support. It will be of benefit to teachers, therapists, group workers, play workers, midday supervisors and support workers, as well as to parents and siblings of children with autism.

an **informa** business

ISBN 978-0-86388-821-2

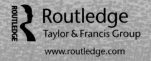

Routledge
Taylor & Francis Group

www.routledge.com